SURGICAL REVOLUTIONS

A Historical and Philosophical View

SURGICAL REVOLUTIONS

A Historical and Philosophical View

Luis H. Toledo-Pereyra

Michigan State University
Kalamazoo Center for Medical Studies
Western Michigan University, USA

World Scientific

NEW JERSEY · LONDON · SINGAPORE · BEIJING · SHANGHAI · HONG KONG · TAIPEI · CHENNAI

Published by

World Scientific Publishing Co. Pte. Ltd.

5 Toh Tuck Link, Singapore 596224

USA office: 27 Warren Street, Suite 401-402, Hackensack, NJ 07601

UK office: 57 Shelton Street, Covent Garden, London WC2H 9HE

British Library Cataloguing-in-Publication Data
A catalogue record for this book is available from the British Library.

ISBN-13 978-981-4329-62-0
ISBN-10 981-4329-62-2

Typeset by Stallion Press
Email: enquiries@stallionpress.com

Printed by FuIsland Offset Printing (S) Pte Ltd. Singapore

To my dear granddaughters
Remington Rose (Remi), Alexandra Avalon (Lexi),
and Elia Sophia
for a life full of love and understanding,
from Papa Lacho

Contents

Contributors

Luis H. Toledo-Pereyra, MD, PhD
Departments of Research and Surgery
Michigan State University/
Kalamazoo Center for Medical Studies
and Department of History
Western Michigan University
Kalamazoo, Michigan, USA
toledo@kcms.msu.edu

Robert M. Langer, MD, PhD
Departments of Surgery and Transplantation
Semmelweis University
Budapest, Hungary
roblanger@hotmail.com

Roberto Anaya-Prado, MD, PhD
Department of Research and Education
Hospital of Obstetrics and Gynecology
Centro Médico de Occidente
Instituto Mexicano del Seguro Social (IMSS)
Guadalajara, Jalisco, México
robana@prodigy.net.mx

Eduardo D. Aceves-Velàzquez, MD, PhD
Department of Research and Education
Hospital of Obstetrics and Gynecology
Centro Médico de Occidente
Instituto Mexicano del Seguro Social (IMSS)
Guadalajara, Jalisco, México

Sara P. Carillo-Cuenca, MD
Department of Research and Education
Hospital of Obstetrics and Gynecology
Centro Médico de Occidente
Instituto Mexicano del Seguro Social (IMSS)
Guadalajara, Jalisco, México

Preface

This book was born from an idea I had on the evolution of surgical history and how a series of surgical revolutions throughout many centuries radically changed the face and expression of the discipline. *Surgical Revolutions* emanated mostly from non-surgically related events that were critically needed to advance the science and better practice of surgery.

Vesalius with his anatomy, Harvey with the recognition of the heart and circulatory physiology, Leeuwenhoek with the detection of small animals through improved microscopy and the introduction of anesthesia by Long and Morton, among others, were the initial discoveries representing the surgical revolutions.

Bernard, Pasteur and Lister completed the next stage of particularly advanced knowledge that created the following phase of *Surgical Revolutions*. Knowledge more than technique represented the fundamental need, since surgeons could operate but had no way to sustain their results.

In 1865 Joseph Lister's (1827-1912) scientific surgery appeared and gained momentum with other surgeon-researchers, who, within one to two decades, began introducing their surgical contributions. The birth of scientific surgery with the advancements of antiseptic surgery marked an unique and profoundly important surgical revolution.

In 1895, at the end of the 19th century, Roentgen, a German physicist, put forward what would be a great discovery for the surgical profession, the use of x-rays. This noted development constituted the last surgical revolution of that century.

Other revolutions in surgery, which are not reported herein, occurred in the following century, such as the commitment to research, the formal development of neurosurgery, vascular surgery, cardiac surgery, transplantation, and most recently, orthopedic, bariatric, laparoscopic and robotic surgery. Other significant events included the discovery of sulfur, heparin, and antibiotics. In addition, parenteral nutrition, improved body imaging, and critical care advances rounded out the 20th century.

It is my sincere wish that this book will enhance your desire to explore further the development and origins of other surgical revolutions, past or present.

Luis H. Toledo-Pereyra, MD, PhD

SECTION I
SURGICAL REVOLUTIONS

Surgical Revolutions

by Luis H. Toledo-Pereyra, MD, PhD

Throughout history, many revolutions in the surgical sciences have occurred. Some are small, others more dominant, but always with the idea of improving the art and science of surgery. In this account we analyze the philosophical understanding of surgical revolutions.

What is a Surgical Revolution Anyhow?

Like any revolution, a surgical revolution represents change, most significantly in the knowledge and practice of surgery. A surgical revolution is the way that colleagues and patients accept new concepts in the evolution of the discipline. A revolution is the different manner by which society incorporates new ideas into the soul of the field. A revolution is a new paradigm demonstrated to be valid when caring for surgical patients.

How do we Recognize a Surgical Revolution?

Recognizing a surgical revolution is a simple process if the revolution is overwhelming in nature and scope, for instance, the introduction of antisepsis by Lister[1] and asepsis by Volkman and von Bergman.[2] These unique contributions are monumental examples of the perspicacity, determination and belief of the individuals behind them.

Just imagine how Lister must have felt while reaching the conclusion that antisepsis was fundamental in the art of curing patients undergoing even the simplest surgical procedures. Just analyze how others persisted to reach the point of no return in the acceptance of their discoveries.

On the other hand, it is difficult to recognize a revolution if it is minor or of diminished significance. We can allude, for example, to the introduction of new surgical instruments, new sutures, etc., which involved incremental change and, therefore, are not as important as the major revolutions that produced fundamental changes.

Are Surgical Revolutionaries Different?

Certainly, surgical revolutionaries have set the pace of the discipline or have opened up new and different roads for others to follow, have indeed contributed a great deal to the specialty, and are different from the day-to-day practitioner who has continued in the path set by others.

Surgical revolutionaries can come in the guises of Lister (antisepsis), Billroth (gastrointestinal surgery), McBurney (appendicitis), Kocher (thyroid surgery), Halsted (surgical residency and safe surgery), Cushing (safe brain surgery), Wangensteen (gastrointestinal physiological surgery), Blalock (relief of cyanotic heart disease), Lillehei (open heart surgery), and many others.

Surgical revolutionaries can also appear in the likes of Carrel (vascular anastomoses and organ transplantation), Forssman (cardiac catheterization), Huggins (hormonal effect in cancer), Graham (oral cholecystography and lung cancer), Gibbons (heart-lung machine), Murray (successful live-twin kidney transplant), and many others.

And surgical revolutionaries can also emerge as did DeBakey (arterial reconstruction, heart pump), Starzl (liver transplantation), Najarian (kidney transplants), Buchwald (surgical treatment of obesity and cholesterol), Shires (fluid management after trauma), and many others.

What are the Qualities of Surgical Revolutionaries?

Surgical revolutionaries have many qualities in common with surgical innovators and surgical discoverers. For instance, all three groups possess the initiative to discover, innovate or to revolutionize; all three have the commitment and determination to succeed; all three have the perseverance to stay focused on the task at hand. Now, the differences among the three surface in their overall goals. The revolutionary is making a change, the innovator is introducing a modification to a well-known principle or technique, and the discoverer is initiating a completely new idea or way of treatment.

Surgical revolutionaries are leading the surgical community and establishing the pace of evolution in surgery. They are the leaders of the school of new advances in surgery. They are changing the way of practice!

Is There a Way to Educate the New Surgical Revolutionaries?

Of course there is, in the same way that we can educate surgical innovators and surgical discoverers. The main consideration will be to establish an effective curriculum which represents the ideas and principles of a surgical revolution. That is conceptualizing the knowledge and practice of surgery, knowing what is available and how deficiencies could be improved upon, how the concept of change, innovation or discovery could be taught in theory and practice.

Emerging surgical revolutionaries should receive a well-structured plan that permits them to recognize means to advance their ideas, their way of thinking, and opportunities to grow and prosper as well. The plan ideally would have deadlines for projects and accomplishments, and would define the best approach to testing the surgical principles and ideas learned, knowing that to revolutionize is to change the paradigms currently governing surgery.

Can History Provide Long Lasting Examples of Surgical Revolutions?

Definitely, the history of surgery provides us with a long list of examples that could very well support the learning of the principles associated with a surgical revolution. History would bring the principal actors, would discuss the roads they follow to create a surgical revolution, and would establish the characteristics of change previously addressed.

With the hindsight of history we can recognize patterns of progress, evaluate means of advancing a new cause, and in this way solidify details of innovative behavior that could lead to a surgical revolution.

Let's take for example Owen Wangensteen (1898–1981), the great American surgeon-leader from a Minnesota farm who reached the heights of medical science at the University of Minnesota and beyond to the rest of the world. He introduced revolutionary concepts in stomach and bowel decompression, he considered second-look abdominal re-operation as a way to assess the progression of ovarian cancer, among other advances, and he developed a unique surgical school that was second to none in the world. The advanced Minnesota teacher and his disciples provided many surgical revolutions during his lifetime. Thus, history offers us the opportunity to learn from surgical revolutionaries such as Owen Wangensteen.

Are There Different Kinds of Surgical Revolutions?

Yes, indeed. Many surgical revolutions of different kinds exist. They can be major, minor, or in between. Major revolutions, for example, include the antiseptic surgical revolution, the aseptic surgical revolution, the x-ray revolution, the safe surgery revolution, the surgical residency revolution, the abdominal surgery revolution, and a cadre of unparalleled revolutions that excited the mind and stimulated the practice of surgical specialists.[3–5] Well into the 20th century, other revolutions occupied the attention of surgical revolutionaries and common surgeons as well.

Minor revolutions in surgery include those instituted daily by the surgeon who changes a type of suture, uses a different incision, opens or closes the surgical wound differently, modifies excision of a tumor, or introduces a slew of other changes in operating rooms around the world.

Surgeons can be revolutionaries if they are amenable to improving the outcome of their patients by making a change that is effective and well thought out through any of the phases of the process — pre-, intra-, and post-operatively. All surgeons can be agents of change, can be revolutionaries, and can improve the practice of surgery.

Evaluating Surgical Revolutions Within the Context of Science and Technology

Connor[3] from the National Museum of Health and Medicine at the Armed Forces Institute of Pathology in Washington, D.C., has advanced an interesting concept, namely that "the components of the surgical revolution are grounded in techniques and medical devices — innovations that, at heart, are technological."[3] A surgical revolution is then primarily technology-based according to Connor. Even though this assertion is highly suggestive and truthful in essence, other factors, such as the science behind revolutions, can be dominant and sometimes unique as the source of change. It is realistic to think that technology can drive science or, vice versa, that science can propel technological change. In the end, both of them, science and technology, participate in the surgical revolution, sometimes more one than the other, but both always present.

Basalla,[6] a well respected technology expert, very astutely indicated that "technology is not the servant of science." He proposed a middle way between science and technology, and I would add that both have a great deal to contribute to the advancement of a surgical revolution. Technology is art or craft and science is the systematic study of a specific event, phenomenon or function. Understanding science and technology will better define their roles in the development of a surgical revolution.

Science and technology, both, are at the core of determining whether surgical revolutions succeed or fail. In this sense, surgical revolutionaries need to promote and only accept superior science and technology. The more understood and tested the new methods and techniques applied to surgery, the more consistent and worthwhile the surgical revolution will be.

Are There New Surgical Revolutions Worth Considering Today?

Many advances in surgery have occurred in the past few decades. Aside from the revolutions of open heart surgery, transplantation, metabolic surgery, scan-guided surgical techniques, precise excision of brain-localized pathology and others, robotic surgery stands as one of the most recent important surgical revolutions.

Robotic surgery is a technological and scientific advance that has convinced the medical and lay community of its efficacy and practicality. Surgeons and patients alike have seen the immediate advantages of techniques utilizing robotic surgery. The outreach of these procedures is enormous, with demonstrated benefit for patients who remain hospitalized for shorter periods of time and return to work in a prompt and productive manner.

Conclusion

Surgical revolutions have appeared throughout history in an uneven manner and strictly based on the scientific and technological knowledge available at the time of the revolution. Great personalities behind a surgical revolution are evidently a significant force dealing with the completion of the event. A combination of commitment, perseverance and availability of science and technology are required elements in the road to a surgical revolution. Innovation and discovery can hasten the progress of a revolutionary event. The better understanding and complete analysis of surgical revolutions would allow our fellow surgeons to be more aware of the concepts and ideas and to participate in future revolutions.

References

1. Toledo-Pereyra LH, Toledo MM. (1976) A critical study of Lister's work on antiseptic surgery. *Mer J Surg* **131**:736–744.
2. Toledo-Pereyra LH, Toledo MM. (1979) Anticontagionism in the opposition to Lister. *Curr Surg* **36**:78–87.
3. Connor JTH. (2004) Beyond the ivory tower: the Victorian revolution in surgery. *Science* **304**:54 (available at www.sciencemag.org/cgi/content/full304).
4. Crowther MA, Dupree MW. (2007) *Medical Lives in the Age of Surgical Revolution.* Cambridge University Press, Cambridge.
5. Youngson AJ. (1979) *The Scientific Revolution in Victorian Medicine.* Holmes & Meier, New York.
6. Basalla G. (1988) *The Evolution of Technology. History of Science.* Cambridge University Press, Cambridge.

2

De Humani Corporis Fabrica
Surgical Revolution

by Luis H. Toledo-Pereyra, MD, PhD

Surgery would not have matured as it has without the seminal anatomical contributions of Andreas Vesalius (1514–1564), without the new way of presenting anatomy to the surgical and medical world, without the surgical revolution that emanated from *De Humani Corporis Fabrica*, published in 1543.[1]

Andreas Vesalius took anatomy in all its complexity and transformed it into an incredible and interesting new medical discipline by systematically arranging and illustrating bones, muscles, veins, arteries, organs, and their intricate interrelationships. Vesalius created a surgical revolution when he introduced *De Humani Corporis Fabrica* to the entire universe of medicine and surgery. Our intention is to decipher the most important elements associated with this extraordinary revolution.

Anatomy Before Galen

From legendary times, Greek physicians considered anatomy as a worthwhile aspect of medical knowledge.[2] Alcmaeon of Crotona (~500 BC) in southern Italy began dissecting animals (mainly goats) before anyone else, and stated that the brain was an essential organ of intelligence.[3]

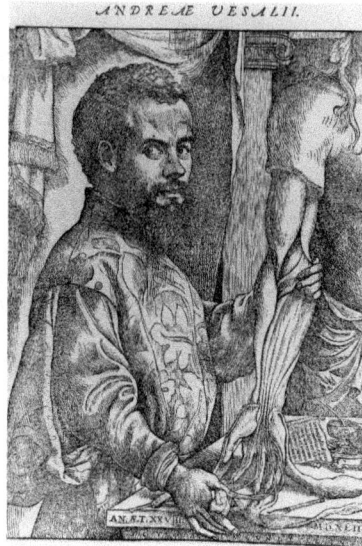

Figure 2.1.   Picture of Vesalius, age 28.

Hippocrates and his disciples followed in the fifth century BC. They noted the significance of bones, joints, and other important structures.

Aristotle (384–322 BC) preferred the study of zoology over the characterization of anatomy in animals. He never performed human dissection, in spite of which his findings were applied to humans. He was a biologist with some commitment to anatomy. Aristotle never practiced medicine or surgery. His contributions to anatomy, however, could be summarized in this manner: he discovered two large vessels arising from the heart, even though he did not name them and the description of the vein was incomplete; and he separated the trachea from the esophagus, identified the epiglottis and larynx, and recognized some of the structures of the lung. Wrongly, he attributed three ventricles to the human heart. Aristotle considered the heart to be the center of life and emotion, putting him at odds with others who considered the brain to be such a center.[2–4]

Deocles of Carystos (384–322 BC) continued in the tradition of Aristotle and attended Athens Dogmatic School. It is not known if he performed some human dissection, but he first utilized the word "anatomy."[2] Praxogoras of Cos followed Diocles, and was the first to distinguish a vein from an artery. Erroneously, he felt the arteries carried pneuma (air), and believed that they were transformed into nerves when diminished in size.[2]

The gifted Hellenistic School of anatomy was next. Herophilus of Chalcedon (335–280 BC) and Erasistratus of Iulis (304–250 BC) were its main protagonists. Herophilus undertook human dissection for the first time in history,[2] and can be considered the father of anatomy. He corrected Aristotle and Praxogoras, and eliminated the Aristotelian thinking that the heart was of central importance to the human body; instead he believed the brain to be at this juncture.[2] He recognized the differences between motor and sensory nerves, described the cerebrum and cerebellum, encountered the optic nerves, followed them, and described the *rete mirabile* (later determined by Vesalius to be present only in animals.[2] Many more accomplishments were attributed to Herophilus: the recognition of the pulse and its possible relationship to the heart; the identification of the venous artery and arterial vein of the pulmonary circulation; the naming of the duodenum; and the description of the Fallopian tubes were testimony to his extraordinary insights.[2,4]

Erasistratus, however, focused more on physiology and the cardiovascular system. He recognized the cardiac valves, even though Hippocrates had mentioned them before.[2] "In diastole, the heart expanded, blood was drawn into the right ventricle whence it passed to the lung to nourish it," said O'Malley when describing the contributions of Erasistratus. Furthermore, the pneuma (air) was breathed into the lung, the left ventricle, the arteries, and the rest of the body "to provide vitality" ("vital spirit") according to Erasistratus.[2]

The study of human anatomy was halted in Alexandria around 150 BC,[2] and dedicated interest in anatomy turned to the Roman Empire.[2] Celsus (25 BC–50 AD) was an erudite Roman writer, who compiled *De Medicina* as an encyclopedia that included references to diet, pharmacy, and surgery.[2–4] References to anatomy were limited, since his work was mainly clinical. Another noted anatomist of the pre-Galenic period was Rufus of Ephesus (between the last century BC and the first century AD), whose studies were on animals and described a four-to-five lobed liver. His findings were frequently applied to humans and mistakenly attributed to Galen.[2]

Anatomy of Galen

The genius of Galen focused on exploring and defining the anatomical structures encountered in the animals (usually Barbary apes) utilized in his experiments. Galen was precise and detailed in his approach, and driven to accomplish the best in his studies. However, according to George Corner, noted anatomist from the University of Rochester, "Galen was not very systematic, he was repetitious, inconsistent and at the same time very positive in matters of opinion."[3] Galen embodied a different approach than the surgeons and physicians of antiquity, who were oriented toward and committed to understanding the principles of the science of the day.[2-5]

Galen produced many excellent works of anatomy, beginning with *On Anatomical Procedures*. Another important work was *On Bones for Beginners*, in which he categorized bones as long bones or flat bones.[5] Galen identified apophyses and epiphyses. Trochanter came from another source.[5] He accurately described vertebrae, ribs, sternum, clavicle, and the bones of the limbs.[5] The bones of the skull, and 24 vertebrae with the coccyx and sacrum were well described too.[5] Diarthrosis and synarthrosis were also recognized by Galen.[5]

The description of the muscular system represented the jewel of Galen's works.[5] His book, *On the Anatomy of the Muscles*, depicted the most accurate analysis available for its time.[5] According to Singer,[5] a notable historian of Greek medicine, one barrier during these times was the absence of a complete anatomical nomenclature, particularly for the muscles, bones, nerves and related structures.

Galen identified seven cranial nerves[4,5] compared to the 12 we know today. The optic nerve was the first, the oculomotor and abducent the second, the trigeminal the third and fourth, the facial auditory the fifth, the glossopharyngeal, vagus and spinal the sixth, and the hypoglossal the seventh.[4,6] Galen recognized the sympathetic system and traced part of it.[6] Many of the structures of the brain, such as the corpus callosum, the corpora quadrigemina, the fornix, the pineal body, and the septum pellucidum were characterized by the master of anatomy.[4] The recurrent laryngeal nerves were well-identified as well.[5]

In his work, *On the Anatomy of the Veins and Arteries*, Galen indicated that the arteries came from the heart and the veins from the liver.[4,5] The angiology of Galen was not as advanced as his osteology and myology.[5] In other works, Galen described the organs of the reproductive system, fetal development, and other structures of the body.[4,5] Galen introduced physiology in addition to his anatomic descriptions. Not surprisingly, the accomplished surgeon of the gladiators[7] brought well-deserved recognition to Pergamon, his natal city, and to Greece, his accepted country. The celebrated anatomist reached fame and respect in the world of medical antiquity because of his unsurpassed contributions to anatomy and surgery.[7]

Anatomy After Galen and Before Vesalius

With the death of Galen in 200 AD, Greek science began a steady decline and the Dark Ages opened the door to an incredible stagnation in the intellectual life of Europe and the Western world. According to Corner, "Anatomy seems to have disappeared completely; no book on the subject is known to have been in use in Europe before the 12th century, except a trivial fragment of Vindician, preserved in the Beneventan script of southern Italy."[3]

Islamic dominance in science occurred from the eighth to the 13th centuries when "the most important documents of Greek medicine were translated into Arabic."[5] These works were then translated into Latin and disseminated to the world. The unique translating work of Constantine the African (d. 1087), in South Italy in the monastery of Monte Cassimo, is worth mentioning. Stephen of Antioch and Gerard of Cremona (1115–1185) were two other recognized translators.[4,5] It is interesting to note that the best known Arabic physician writers — Avicenna, Hali Abbas and Rhazes — depended for their anatomy on Galen's Arabic versions.[5] The influence of the Pergamon surgeon and anatomist is clear.

William of Saliceto (and Henri of Mondeville) utilized Aristotle's, Galen's and Avicenna's anatomy works to teach their students. Raimondo de Luzzi (Mondino) became the first anatomy teacher in Bologna in 1306 to use human cadavers to teach dissection. His book *Anathomia*, published in 1316, was dedicated to the study of human dissection and remained the standard text for two centuries.[3–5]

The 14th and 15th centuries saw an increased acceptance of human dissection in public.[3] At first dissection occurred in Italy and then it spread to the rest of Europe.[3] A great personality connected with anatomy at the time was Jacopo Berengario da Carpi (d. 1550). According to Corner,[3] Berengario was the first independent anatomical investigator of modern times. He challenged Galen on many counts, such as the existence of a multi-chambered uterus, the middle ventricle of the heart, and the presence of the *rete mirabile*.[3] By his own account, he offered better descriptions of the heart, brain and larynx.[3]

Anatomy of Vesalius. The Birth of a Surgical Revolution

When *De Humani Corporis Fabrica* appeared in 1543, Vesalius presented to the world a classic of universal literature and to the world of medicine and surgery, in particular, a book that changed both disciplines forever. No other previously published medical book had a similar effect on the evolution of surgery. *De Humani Corporis Fabrica* introduced a great deal of information and precise knowledge regarding the structure of the human body. This book represented a new paradigm, a new way to see human anatomy, a novel and elegant presentation of the human condition.

Vesalius frequently thanked his teacher, Jacobus Sylvius (1478–1555), the first professor in France who utilized human dissection in his anatomy class, and from whom he learned dissection techniques and the teachings of Galen.[6] Sadly, after the publication of Vesalius' book, their friendship became adversarial, and Sylvius, "filled with jealousy and rage, became vindictive."[6] In spite of this development, Vesalius knew that he owed a great deal to his teacher and that Sylvius would be one of the individuals to whom Vesalius would always be indebted. In some ways, Sylvius was an early part of the initial stages of the anatomical revolution by just being Andreas Vesalius' teacher, even though they ended up in opposite camps.

From the University of Paris, Vesalius moved in 1539 to the University of Padua, which was considered "one of the great intellectual centers of Europe."[4] On December 6, 1537, one day after Vesalius received his Doctor of Medicine, he was appointed Professor of Surgery and the first chair in Anatomy. According to professor Persaud, "Vesalius was supremely successful as a teacher because of his skill as a dissector and his enthusiastic expositions and demonstrations, which he personally carried out. Indeed, his greatest innovation as an anatomist was that he dissected corpses himself and lectured at the same time."[4] His course was popular and well attended.

Vesalius prepared *De Humani Corporis Fabrica* after several years of dedicated study and innumerable human dissections. Detailed observation, careful analysis of anatomical facts, and the extraordinary help of an artist of the magnitude of Jan Calcar, and probably of other art students of the Titian school, culminated in a unique book of human anatomy — the best ever to be assembled!

Johannes Oporinus (1507–1568), publisher and scholar in Basel, received the book and the wood blocks for final printing in late 1542. Vesalius personally supervised the production of the book.[4] The results were obvious to the medical world. A great scientific and artistic compendium was the end product — a book that was going to modify the way future students observed and studied anatomy.

Vesalius had the courage to pursue his convictions. He believed in what he had seen while performing human dissections. He stated his findings aloud for the scientific and world communities to hear. Persaud put it in this way: "The publication of Vesalius' *De Humani Corporis Fabrica* in 1543 ushered in a new era in the history of medicine and marked the beginning of modern anatomy. The work emanated from an analytical mind who knew that in order to describe the true structure of the human body he had to first dissect it. Vesalius' observations were not always in agreement with the established teachings of Galen, which were slavishly accepted for more than 12 centuries. Nevertheless, he had the courage to describe what he saw, for in science lies only truth."[6]

Why did this book create a surgical revolution? Many reasons support this strong assertion. The first reason relates to the accurate and extensive information that Vesalius gave surgeons in the practice of the profession. Second, good surgery without good anatomy is not feasible. Advances in surgery are frequently dependent on advances in anatomy, which are simultaneously associated with good and precise anatomical descriptions, such as the ones in *De Humani Corporis Fabrica*. Third, this book offered a new direction for the practicing surgeon, who was searching for new avenues of knowledge to advance the surgical field. Fourth, Vesalius made it easier for the surgeon to become familiar with the intricacies of human anatomy. Before this work, there were no consistent treatises that clearly presented anatomy, specifically not in a manner of the Belgian master.

In conclusion, *De Humani Corporis Fabrica* created a surgical revolution because no other book or publication had ever influenced surgeons in the way this book did. For all this, Vesalius should be considered a surgical revolutionary as well.

References

1. Sherzoi H. (2005) Andreas Vesalius. In: LH Toledo-Pereyra (ed.). *Vignettes on Surgery, History and Humanities*. Landes Bioscience, Georgetown, TX.
2. O'Malley CD. (1964) *Andreas Vesalius of Brussels 1514–1564*. University of California Press, Berkeley, CA.
3. Corner GW. (1964) *Anatomy*. Hafner Publishing Company, New York.
4. Persaud TVN. (1984) *Early History of Human Anatomy*. Charles C. Thomas Publishers, Springfield, IL.
5. Singer C. (1957) *A Short History of Anatomy and Physiology from the Greeks to Harvey*. Dover Publications Inc., New York.
6. Persaud TVN. (1997) *A History of Anatomy. The Post-Vesalian Era*. Charles C. Thomas Publishers, Springfield, IL.
7. Toledo-Pereyra LH. (2002) Claudius Galenus of Pergamon: surgeon of gladiators. Father of experimental physiology. *J Invest Surg* **15**(6):299–301.

3

Exercitatio Anatomica de Motus Cordis et Sanguinis in Animalibus Surgical Revolution

by Luis H. Toledo-Pereyra, MD, PhD

William Harvey (1578–1657) has been well-known for several centuries in the most exclusive confines of medicine and surgery as the father of circulation. Harvey's comprehensive and innovative approach to the understanding of the circular path of the circulation of the blood made him the unique medical hero we know today.[1–12]

Harvey's ideas widely expressed in his classic book *Exercitatio Anatomica De Motus Cordis et Sanguinis in Animalibus* (1628), represented a completely new direction in the understanding of the physiology of the heart and its circulation.[6–8] The enormous implications of his work on the cardiovascular, transplant, and vascular surgery of our day constituted a surgical revolution of incredible proportions. *De Motus Cordis,* as we call it in its abbreviated form, is the premier writing of Harvey's revolution. Our work focuses its attention onto the extraordinary preludes and actual discovery of the circulation by this gifted English physician.

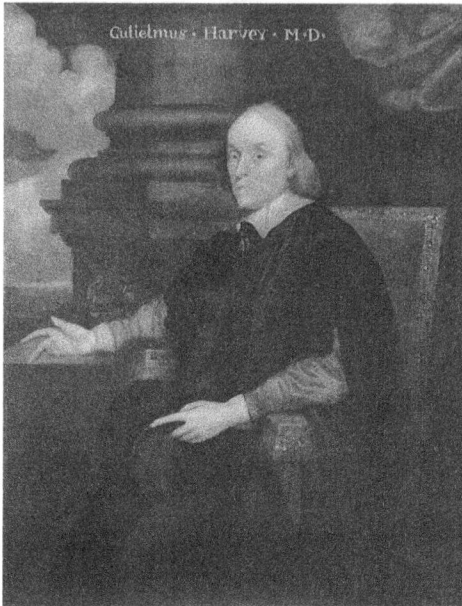

WILLIAM HARVEY
Royal College of Physicians

Figure 3.1.   Painted portrait of Harvey.

Cardiovascular Work Before Galen

Many ideas related to the anatomy and function of the heart were introduced by physicians before Galen (129–200 AD), who practiced in the second century. Five hundred years before Galen, Aristotle (384–322 BC), the great philosopher, biologist, and ethicist was the leading candidate among aspiring anatomists or morphologists of his epoch.

In the fifth century BC, the Greek medical writer Empedocles from Sicily believed that the heart was at the center of "pneuma" and the vascular system.[1] Diogenes of Apollonia, around the same time, declared the importance of the blood vessels.[1] Hippocratic writers, also around the fifth century BC, did not advance the medical knowledge on the heart or the vascular tree further than previous medical contributors. In the pre-Christian fourth century, Diocles, practicing in Athens, considered the heart an essential organ and the seat of intelligence as well.[1]

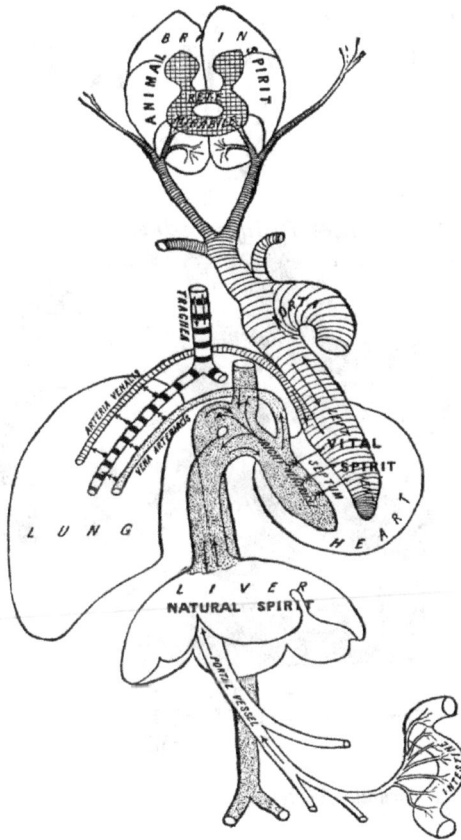

Figure 3.2.   Diagram of Galen's cardiovascular system research.

Aristotle, the noted Greek academician, supported the heart as the center of organ primacy and recognized branches of the vena cava and superficial vessels of the arm.[1] He assigned three chambers to the heart and identified the *ductus arteriosus*. He also proposed that the arteries usually ran along veins.[1] Aristotle, however, did not assign great importance to the brain.[1]

Now we move quickly to the great Alexandrians Herophilus of Chalcedon (around 300 BC), named "Father of Anatomy," and Erasistratus of Keos (325–250 BC), named "Father of Physiology," to pay tribute to their extraordinary contributions on the refined anatomy and physiology

ᕮXᕮRCITATIO
ANATOMICA DE
MOTV CORDIS ET SAN-
GVINIS IN ANIMALI-
BVS,

GVILIELMI HARVEI ANGLI,
Medici Regii, & Profefforis Anatomiæ in Col-
legiæ Medicorum Londinenfi.

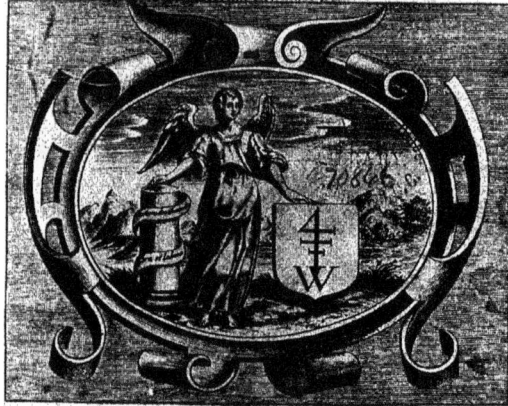

FRANCOFVRTI,
Sumptibus GVILIELMI FITZERI.
ANNO M. DC. XXVIII.

Figure 3.3.   *Exercitatio Anatomica* book cover, as published in 1628.

of the past.[1,13] The Chalcedonian did not attach as much significance to the heart as he did to the brain, which he designated as the seat of intelligence, antagonizing in this point the great Aristotle.[1] He established a clear distinction between arteries and veins, and defined pulsation in a more specific manner as originating from arteries themselves.[1] The Keos physiologist took the level of cardiovascular knowledge to the highest position ever when he regarded the heart as the source of both arteries and veins, far ahead of any contemporary and ahead of anyone else until Harvey.[1] Erasistratus also identified a communication system between arteries and veins, which later became the well-known capillary system.

Erasistratus made unique contributions in describing the atrioventricular valves, their functional purpose and the chorda tendineae as well.[4] The semilunar valves had been described before in *De Corde*, one of the possible late Hippocratic writings.[4]

Cardiovascular Work During Galen's Time

The genius of Galen permeated the medical scene and controlled medicine and surgery for 1400 years. Master Galen could not be right all the time! In fact, several errors were detected in some of his discoveries. Many believed the errors stemmed from extrapolating his work from animals to humans.

In the cardiovascular system, the surgeon of the gladiators, the great Greek-Roman physician, described the valves again, differentiated arteries and veins, and demonstrated, contrary to many of his predecessors, that the arteries contained and carried blood and not "pneuma."[14] He wrongly believed that small interventricular pores allowed for the passage of blood from the right to the left heart.[4] Galen considered the heart not as a pump, but rather as a sucking system obtaining the blood from the veins.[14]

Galen considered two types of blood, the "nutritive blood" made in the liver and carried through veins, and the "vital blood" made by the heart and carried through arteries.[14]

Cardiovascular Discoveries After Galen

No worthwhile discoveries regarding the heart or the vascular system — including the works of Avicenna (930–1022 BC) — occurred after Galen's time in the second century until the appearance of Ibn-al-Nafis (1213–1288) during the high Middle Ages. He studied medicine in Damascus, Syria, where he had been born, and in El Cairo where he finished his medical schooling.[4]

Today, Ibn-al-Nafis is considered the discoverer of pulmonary circulation.[4] It is quite remarkable that without known anatomical dissections or well-confirmed experimental studies, he conceived the pulmonary circulation from Galen's observations and his own innovative thinking.[4] Ibn-al-Nafis was the most advanced physician and scholar of his times. He delved into many areas of human endeavor that took him far beyond medicine. He was a lawyer, theologian, philosopher, astronomer, linguist, and historian, besides being a physician and surgeon.[15]

The full demonstration of the pulmonary circulation can be clearly traced to one of Ibn-al-Nafis' superb writings, a "Commentary on Anatomy in Avicenna's Canon":[15]

> "...the blood from the right chamber of the heart must arrive at the left chamber but there is no direct pathway between them. The thick septum of the heart is not perforated and does not have visible pores as some people thought or invisible pores as Galen thought. The blood from the right chamber must flow through the vena arteriosa (pulmonary artery) to the lungs, spread through its substances, be mingled there with air, pass through the arteria venosa (pulmonary vein) to reach the left chamber of the heart and there form the vital spirit...."

In another portion of Ibn-al-Nafis' descriptions, he indicated:[15,16]

> "The heart has only two ventricles...and between these two there is absolutely no opening. Also dissection gives this lie to what they said, as the septum between these two cavities is much thicker than elsewhere. The benefit of this blood (that is in the right cavity) is to go up to the lungs, mix with what is in the lungs of air, then pass through the arteria venosa to the left cavity of the two cavities of the heart... ."

Around the same time as the noted Arabic writings of Ibn-al-Nafis, a great number of European surgeons, anatomists and writers dedicated themselves to the study of anatomical concepts and ideas. Hugh da Lucca (1170–1240) and Theodoric Borgognoni (1205–1298) from the Surgical School at Bologna, William of Saliceto (1215–1280?), also a Bolognese surgeon who completed his surgery book in 1275, and Thaddeus of Florence (1223–1303) were credible precursors of the advanced anatomy of the times.[1] Henri de Mondeville (1270–1320) followed Thaddeus but did not add much to what was already known at the time. Mondino da Luzzi (1270–1326) was the last of this group of respected anatomists and himself had been a disciple of Thaddeus as well. In total, the anatomical descriptions of these surgeons-anatomists-writers were not new in the cardiovascular arena, and basically they subscribed to the entire Galenic-Avicennian principles without taking significant steps towards the future of this discipline. Even the French surgeon Guy de Chauliac (1300–1370), and later on the Italians anatomical professors Gabriele da Gerbi (died 1505) and Alessandro Achillini (1463–1512), did not earn any praises for their cardiovascular knowledge or advances thereof.[1]

Cardiovascular Work of Leonardo, Vesalius, Servetus and Colombo

The extraordinary period of the Renaissance (1453–1600s?) opened up a new and exciting era of medical advances. Individuals with fresh and innovative thinking immediately appeared on the horizon. Among them, Leonardo da Vinci (1452–1519) presented particularly unique ideas in the world of science and anatomy, among many other disciplines in which he showed his sheer genius.

The printing press was assembled for the first time in 1440, creating a new vehicle for disseminating knowledge. This innovation brought about its own scientific revolution. Leonardo and many of the scholars of the time utilized the benefits of the printing press by publishing all their advanced writings.[4,7,12]

da Vinci made a great number of contributions to the cardiovascular field, most of them, however, were a confirmation of previous works and not well-defined discoveries. He developed experiments to demonstrate the action of the valves and the movement of the heart.[1] According to Key and associates,[4] da Vinci thought of the heart as a pump and understood the synchronicity of the pulse and heartbeat.

Andreas Vesalius (1514–1564) came next and essentially changed the face of anatomy, generating a true surgical revolution, more than had ever been accomplished before. Vesalius single handedly put anatomy on the medical map. His advances in the cardiovascular area were consistent with the improved knowledge that originated from performing numerous human dissections. Vesalius carefully participated in the drawing of the arterial and venous systems as well as the heart. He thoroughly described the anatomy of all these important structures and also recognized that the blood did not go from the right to the left ventricle. He did not encounter pores in the interventricular septa, as Galen had suggested before. Vesalius made an indelible mark in the history of anatomy and, therefore, in the history of surgery and medicine.

Michael Servetus (1511–1553) followed Vesalius in terms of time but not in geographical origin. Servetus hailed from the province of Aragon in Spain, where he embraced the Catholic religious life as well as medicine. In spite of his controversial religious ideas on the dogma of the Trinity, which cost him his life for heresy under Calvin, Servetus excelled in medical anatomical knowledge and in the description of pulmonary circulation.[4] In 1553, his great book, *Christianismi Restitutio*, was published. In it Servetus advanced the status of the circulation by fully recognizing that the blood would leave the right ventricle, go to the lungs, and then move to the left ventricle, in this way completing the whole pulmonary vascular circuit.

Realdo Colombo (1516–1559), of Italian descent, followed Vesalius at the University of Padua where he was appointed as his successor.[12] After several years, he moved to Venice and then to Rome where he became a professor at the University La Sapienza. Colombo did not see his outstanding book, *De re Anatomica*, published since it came to light in 1559, the same year that he passed. In his great work, Colombo described very clearly the pulmonary circulation, based on clinical and experimental studies.[4,12] He studied the heart during diastole and systole, advanced the notion of a one-way mechanism for valve function, and defined the heart muscle contractility and other important anatomical findings.[5,6,9] He continued to believe, however, in several of the anatomical Galenic concepts, such as the presence of intraventricular septum pores and the origin of the pulmonary artery as arising from the liver.

Hieronymus Fabricius (1537–1619), another great Italian anatomist, followed Gabriele Fallopius (1523–1562) at the University of Padua. Fallopius had followed another great Paduan anatomist, Realdo Colombo, who a few years before had taken over the chair of the extraordinary Vesalius. Fabricius' outstanding discovery of the existence of valves in the veins opened the door for Harvey to establish the principles of the circulation of the blood on firm footing.

With the appearance of Fabricuis' notable book, *De Venarum Ostiolis* published in 1603, he completely changed the world of medicine and surgery without realizing the import of his contribution. Fabricius created a surgical revolution when he announced the presence of membranous folds in the veins, which he called valves.[3-5] Even though these structures had been described by other anatomists, including Vesalius, the real contribution of Fabricius was the discovery of a system of valves in all veins of the extremities.[4,11,12] This unique finding not only permitted Harvey to confirm his theory of the circulation of the blood, but advanced the knowledge of the venous system to the point of being helpful to those surgeons who centuries later would anatomically correct the venous pathology.

The Times and Accomplishments of William Harvey — The Creator of a Surgical Revolution

William Harvey had no equals in the world of scientific medicine. He came from England, where he was born in 1578, studied at Caius College in Cambridge, followed by medical school studies at Padua under Fabricius, and graduated in 1602. With all his new knowledge, anatomical concerns and unsatisfied scientific curiosity, he returned to his native country. While in England, he received another doctor of medicine degree from Cambridge. In 1604 he married Elizabeth, the daughter of Lancelot Browne, physician to Queen Elizabeth and James I.[10] Harvey eventually became physician to James I and Charles I.[10]

England presented to Harvey a good opportunity he could not refuse. Memberships to the best medical societies, hospitals and fellowships were attained by him. In 1615, Harvey secured the Lumleian Lecturer position sponsored by the Royal College of Physicians.[4,10,11] This position allowed him to maintain a status of respect in the medical community for the 41 years during which he occupied this prestigious lectureship.[4,11] The inquisitiveness and intense desire of Harvey to understand the physiological problems of the day were quite evident. Harvey approached each problem with sharp and focused intellectual force.

Harvey on the Heart and Circulation of the Blood

There is no evidence that Harvey had begun to conceive his monumental work on the circulation of the blood while he was in Padua. There is no question, however, that he knew about the valves in the veins from his teacher and respected mentor Fabricius while in Italy. At that time, the true meaning of the function of the valves had not been fully determined.[4–6,11,12]

Harvey's own investigations did not begin until his return to England and more specifically to London. When did he start wondering about the circulatory pathway of the blood and motion of the heart? It is hard to know, but the concepts must have been forming between 1604 when he settled in London and 1616 when he began delivering the first Lumleian lectures.[4,11] From Harvey's notes, kept in the British Museum, Key and his group[4] indicated that by 1616 the English scientist had done research on more than 80 types of animals and had begun developing his own theories. Thereafter, Harvey swiftly moved ahead with his ideas pertaining to the heart and circulation of the blood.

By 1616 Harvey began to confirm many important cardiovascular concepts. First, he agreed with previous Colombo findings in that "contraction was the active movement of the heart during which the apex beat occurred and that the systole of the heart coincided with the diastole of the arteries."[11] Second, Harvey confirmed Colombo's ideas regarding the pulmonary circulation, namely that the blood from the right side of the heart traveled via the pulmonary artery, lungs and pulmonary veins to reach the left side of the heart.[11] Third, the significance of the heart valves became evident to Harvey within the context of the movement of blood.[11]

Years later, and according to Whitteridge[11] between 1619 and 1625, Harvey more completely recognized the importance of valves in the veins as a way to explain the movement of the blood in a circle. This is as close as we can approximate in understanding Harvey's evolution to the full discovery of the circulation of the blood. Now, let's proceed with the monumental publication of William Harvey.

De Motu Cordis Published in 1628

Sixteen twenty-eight is the year of the publication of one of the great books of medicine, the book that revolutionized the way that physicians and surgeons thought about the circulation of blood. Previous bits and pieces of knowledge highlighted various aspects of the circulation, but no one realized or discovered the entire movement of the circulation of the blood earlier. Harvey reached the conclusion, that the blood moves in a circular manner, after innumerable experimental and clinical observations and, of course, after analyzing the previous findings of the science of circulation made before him.

Harvey's classic treatise of medical knowledge, *Exercitatio Anatomica de Motu Cordis et Sanguinis in Animalibus* (1628), opened a new era in scientific medicine, established a new paradigm in the confines of anatomy and physiology, and created a revolution in experimental medicine and surgery. This was the book of the century or, better yet, the book of the centuries, the book that transformed the way physicians and surgeons would think about medicine in the future. Harvey studied the motion of the heart and the circulation of the blood with such a patient and thoroughly analytical mind that he convinced most of the medical world with his well-established conclusions. Harvey emerged as the medical investigator par excellence.

Many sections of Harvey's *De Motu Cordis* might be helpful to the avid reader in understanding this unique medical genius. One such passage is quoted by Persaud,[12] who presents Harvey's concluding paragraphs:

"Now then the last place we may bring our opinion, concerning the circulation of the blood, and propound it to all men. Seeing it is confirm'd by reasons and ocular experiments, that the blood does pass through the lungs and heart by the pulse of the ventricles, and is driven in and sent into the whole body, by the pulse of the ventricles, and is driven in and sent into the whole body, and does creep into the veins and porosities of the flesh, and through them returns from the little veins into the greater, from the circumference to the centre, from whence it comes at last into the *vena cava*, and into the ear of the heart in so great abundance, with so great flux and reflux, from hence through the arteries thither, from thence through the veins hither back again, so that it cannot be furnished by those things which we do take in, and in a far greater abundance, than is competent for nourishment: It must be of necessity concluded that the blood is driven into a round by a circular motion in creatures, and that it moves perpetually; and hence does arise the action and function of the heart, which by pulsation it performs; and lastly, that the motion and pulsation at the heart is the only cause."

Harvey After 1628

Harvey continued as a physician to the court of Charles I. Meanwhile he had his personal medical practice, attended patients at St. Bartholomew's Hospital, was an intricate part of the Royal College of Physicians, performed animal dissections, wrote his observations and prepared lectures.

Harvey was an avid reader and preferred Virgil among the literary masters of the past, and Aristotle and Galen in the world of medicine.[2] Harvey dedicated time to the Natural Sciences; in fact, another one of his own books pertained to *The Generation of Animals*, where generation and development were clearly expressed, and where he suggested all animals were produced out of ova.[2]

In spite of his bouts with gout, Harvey continued to be engaged all his life. During the English Civil War of 1642, his house was robbed and many of his valuable papers were lost. In 1645, he was elected Warden of Merton College at Oxford and resigned a year later because of the political surrender of the city in 1646. Harvey slowly deteriorated in health. The king, his close supporter, was in prison, and three of his brothers had died. Harvey's final years were difficult but he stood firm in spite of his personal and political conditions. On June 3, 1657 a great man of science, medicine, and humanity passed!

The Creation of a Surgical Revolution

The publication of Harvey's *Exercitatio Anatomica de Motu Cordis et Sanguinis in Animalibus* in 1628 constituted a surgical revolution, because many years later it significantly modified the way that surgery was practiced. Without the discovery of the "Motion of the Heart and the Circulation of the Blood," the advances realized in the fields of vascular, cardiovascular, and transplant surgeries would not have been possible.

Understanding how the heart worked, how the blood moved in a continuous circle, how the peripheral venous valves functioned, how the arterial and venous blood were different and yet at some point communicated with each other, and how the heart valves opened and closed in synchrony were all important questions that once answered, as they were by

Harvey, created a new and exciting avenue for research, patient care and surgical discovery. He had created a surgical revolution!

The genius and perseverance of Harvey brought with him the first and most important step of the puzzle in the understanding and recognition of the critical relevance of the circulation of the blood. The motion of the heart, the expelling of blood, its return back to the heart, the role of the venous and heart valves, all integrated into an incredibly well-prepared and organized symphony — the symphony of life, the symphony of perfect circulation.

The surgical sciences would not have been the same without the knowledge contributed by Harvey on the motion of the heart and circulation of blood. Advances in cardiac, vascular and transplant surgeries conceived by surgeon investigators centuries later, were attainable in grand part due to the work of Harvey and his historical contemporaries. Harvey is the star of this unique group of contributors and one who should be labeled as the main protagonist of this revolution, perhaps the central figure of this surgical revolution. Without Harvey no revolution would have occurred!

Conclusions

William Harvey is the father of the circulatory system and now should be considered as one of the main contributors in the creation of a surgical revolution, a revolution that gave us the development of cardiac, vascular and transplant surgeries, and a revolution of enormous magnitude.

References

1. Singer C. (1957) *A Short History of Anatomy and Physiology from the Greeks to Harvey*. Dover Publications Inc., New York.
2. Malloch A. (1929) *William Harvey*. Paul B. Hoeber, Inc., New York.
3. Whitteridge G. (1978) William Harvey on the circulation of the blood and on generation. *Am J Med* **85**:880–890.
4. Key JD, Keys TE, Callahan JA. (1979) Historical development of concept of blood circulation. An anniversary memorial essay to William Harvey. *Am J Cardiol* **43**:1026–1032.

5. Gregory A. (2001) *Harvey's Heart, The Discovery of the Blood Circulation.* Icon Books, Cambridge, England.

6. Harvey W. (1990) *The Circulation of the Blood and Other Writings (Everyman's Classics).* Revised Edition. JM Dent, CE Tuttle (eds). Guernsey Press Co., Channel Islands, England.

7. Boas M. (1962) *The Scientific Renaissance 1450–1630.* Harper Torchbooks, Harper and Row Publications, New York.

8. McMullen ET. (1998) *William Harvey and the Use of Purpose in the Scientific Revolution.* University Press of America, Inc., Lanham, Maryland.

9. Bylebyl JJ. (1979) *William Harvey and His Age.* The Johns Hopkins University Press, Baltimore, Maryland.

10. Keynes G. (1966) *The Life of William Harvey.* Oxford University Press, London.

11. Whitteridge G. (1971) *William Harvey and the Circulation of the Blood.* American Elsevier Publishing Co. Inc., New York.

12. Persaud TVN. (1997) *A History of Anatomy The Post-Vesalian Era.* Charles C. Thomas Publications, Springfield, Illinois.

13. Toledo-Pereyra LH. (2006) *Origins of the Knife: Early Encounters with the History of Surgery.* Landes Bioscience, Georgetown, Texas.

14. Phillips RE Jr. *The Heart and the Circulatory System.* Available at http://www.accessexcellence.org/AE/AEC/CC/heart_background.php. Accessed on August 18, 2008.

15. Available at http://en.wikipedia.org/wiki/Ibn_al-Nafis. Accessed on August 18, 2008.

16. Al-Ghazal SK. (2007) *Ibn al-Nafis and the Discovery of the Pulmonary Circulation.* FSTC Limited, Manchester, United Kingdom.

4

The Strange Little Animals of Antony van Leeuwenhoek — Surgical Revolution

by Luis H. Toledo-Pereyra, MD, PhD

Even without knowing it, Antony van Leeuwenhoek (1632–1723) created a true surgical revolution.[1-8] This revolution had its origins in the recognition, for the first time, of a bunch of "strange little animals"[1] that someday would be demonstrated to harm cells, tissues and human bodies. It was the introduction of improved grinding of lenses that permitted Leeuwenhoek to observe small particles or animals and alert other scientists to the critical importance of this unique discovery. The intricacies of his life and innovative path to being praised in the world of science is presented ahead.

Brief Biographical Note

In the city of Delft in Holland, a poorly educated, non-scientist scaled the highest pinnacle of science and accomplishment. Without formal education Leeuwenhoek, with the aid of his commitment and his ability to grind lenses and utilize them for better observation, clearly demonstrated the important value of determination in a willing and interested mind.

Leeuwenhoek had an unnoticeable youth at Delft. His elementary school was unremarkable and at the age of 16 he moved to Amsterdam to

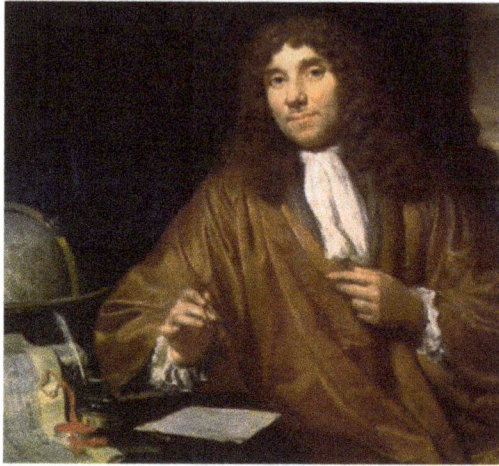

Figure 4.1.   Painted portrait of Leeuwenhoek by artist Jan Verkolje, currently at the Rijksmuseum, The Netherlands (painted between 1670 and 1693, Doek Technique, 56 × 47.5 cm).

follow the business of linen drapery. Six years later, in 1654, he returned to his native city where he set up shop as a draper and married Barbara de Mey, who gave him five children. Unfortunately, she passed in 1666 when Antony was 34 years old[2–5] and their children did not survive to adulthood.

In 1671, he remarried and a child was born from this marriage. This child, Maria, took care of him in his old age, a blessing for this good Dutch worker. Years before, in 1660, Leeuwenhoek had secured a job at the Delft sheriff's office where he worked as a janitor for 39 years.[3] In his spare time and around 1668 he assiduously began to grind glasses and construct microscopes, a long-term secondary profession practiced until the end of his life.[2–5]

Scientific Training

Leeuwenhoek had no scientific training. There were no sites for scientific training at the time. The characterization and definition of modern science had just begun to be conceived by individuals such as Francis Bacon (1561–1626), Robert Hooke (1635–1703), Rene Descartes (1596–1650),

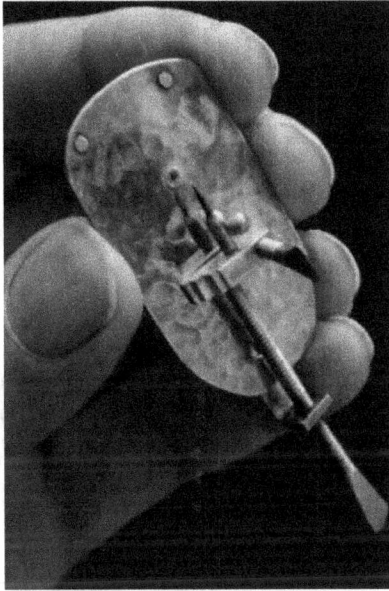

Figure 4.2. Microscope of Leeuwenhoek being held by an unidentified observer. Photograph.

and several other great personalities of the scientific world.[6] Leeuwenhoek was not in that group and never aspired to be included.

His ambition concentrated on seeing "little animals" better and better, for which he had developed better magnifying lenses. His technical processes to grind lenses took him to the center of science during his active microscopic observations. Recognition came from many places in Europe.[2-6]

Even though Leeuwenhoek was not a scientist, his curiosity was unmatched, his skill and diligence were legendary, and his perception of new and unheard of findings was unique. These particular virtues made him a scientist, though he had never trained for the profession. He advanced the field of microscopy to heights never seen before.

The Royal Society

It was Reigner de Graaf, in 1673, who alerted Henry Oldenburg, Secretary of the Royal Society in London, to the extraordinary findings which

Leeuwenhoek was obtaining in Delft with the simple microscope. Immediately thereafter, Oldenburg wrote the uneducated Dutch microscopist for more information, which was fully provided. Thereafter, a long-term association developed and communication successfully ensued with the Royal Society for 50 years.[3,6]

Leeuwenhoek lacked the knowledge of Latin, the language of science in the circles of the Royal Society, and was not able to express his knowledge in English. He wrote all his letters in Dutch. They were presented in a "conversational style" with "random observations" but he never "confused facts with speculations."[3] All his letters were translated into English by instruction of the Royal Society, which cataloged approximately 200 of them.[3]

The Royal Society had great respect for the work and persona of Leeuwenhoek. They admired his findings and committed contributions to the benefit of science. Because of his notable advances in the field of bacteriology and microscopy, he was elected to the Royal Society in 1680,[2-6] a perfectly fitting recognition for the real dedication and discoveries of Leeuwenhoek.

Details of His Observations

From the beginning of his active work with the microscope, Leeuwenhoek never stopped making good and worthwhile contributions to the understanding and improvement of this field of knowledge. His observations were many and varied during a long career that spanned more than 50 years.

Leeuwenhoek discovered a number of bacteria, parasites, cells, fibers, plant tissue, and other material of human tissue and minerals.[6,7] His desire to discover new "little animals" and other yet undescribed tissue or material was insatiable, with no end. His observations carried the sophistication of his commitment, since his scientific education had been limited to only a few years of schooling, completing a maximum of elementary school.

The direct observation of Leeuwenhoek is exemplified by the text of a letter he composed on September 7, 1674. He examined lake water, including the description of the alga spirogyra:

> "Passing just lately over this lake...and examining this water next
> day, I found floating therein divers earthy particles, and some green

streaks, spirally wound serpent-wise, and orderly arranged, after the manner of the copper or tin worms, which distillers use to cool their liquors as they distil over. The whole circumference of each of these streaks was about the thickness of a hair of one's head...all consisted of very small green globules joined together: and there were very many small green globules as well."

In another important descriptive letter, Leeuwenhoek reported on December 25, 1702, about the ciliate organism, *Vorticella*:

"In structure these little animals were fashioned like a bell, and at the round opening they made such a stir, that the particles in the water thereabout were sent in motion thereby...And though I must have seen quite 20 of these little animals on their long tails alongside one another very gently moving, with outstretched bodies and straightened-out tails; yet in an instant, as it were, they pulled their bodies and their tails together, and no sooner had they contracted their bodies and tails, than they began to stick their tails out again very leisurely, and stayed thus some time continuing their gentle motion: which sight I found mightily diverting."

Leeuwenhoek's observations were brought into consideration through his multiple letters sent periodically to the Royal Society. These letters reflected how the draper master and microscopist did not waste any detail in each of his detailed reports.

Life in Science

We already indicated that Leeuwenhoek was not a scientist in the real sense of the word. In spite of that, Leeuwenhoek was able to learn on his own, and I believe his reports constituted the most accurate, scientific, descriptive expression of well-oriented and construed observational research.

The research of Leeuwenhoek was simple, without statistical consideration but directed to report all observable changes, identify all details, and confirm all findings in more than one way.

Without formal education, the Dutch tradesman and microscopist employed a general instinct to be precise and careful in his observations, to the point of having little doubt in the findings reported.

The education of Leeuwenhoek as an amateur scientist came naturally as part of being a meticulous individual, a dedicated describer, and someone who you would trust when analyzing the findings seen under the microscope. Leeuwenhoek and the microscope were a single entity; he understood his lenses, knew how to use them, and how to manage the daily hours spent using the microscope with amazing patience.

Leeuwenhoek's Innovative Work

Leeuwenhoek made significant contributions to the art and knowledge of microscopic advances in the world of biological and technological findings. Here are some of the specific developments:

1. Grinding lenses to be of "exceptional optical quality" and reaching a magnification power of more than 200 diameters,[3-6] when competitors of the stature of Robert Hooke had not reached magnifications of more than 20.
2. Construction of simple microscopes compared to the compound microscopes utilized by Hooke and Swammerdam.[6]
3. Utilization of simple microscopes to make detailed observations of small animals and other living substances and matter.

The actual innovative contributions of Leeuwenhoek can be summarized in two great findings: grinding of lenses and exceptional observational skills. These were the basis for all the advances and improvements accomplished by the unique figure of Leeuwenhoek.

How did He do Everything He did?

This unique human being brought the science of microscopy to the fore when he showed unseen matters to the world of the learned community. No one else had demonstrated what he had done. But how did he do everything?

We do not have a clear answer, even though we think that his accomplishments stemmed from his committed observational ability and his capacity and perseverance in reporting through letters to the Royal Society all of his findings. We think these characteristics joined together to make a successful story for the patient and uneducated Leeuwenhoek, a story to be admired!

Why should Leeuwenhoek's Discoveries be Considered a Surgical Revolution?

A surgical revolution is something that can advance the field of surgery at a given pace. There are small revolutions, medium revolutions and large revolutions. Leeuwenhoek's introduction of the extraordinary opportunity of seeing "strange little animals" under the microscope presented to the surgeon of the future the unique opportunity of identifying surgical infections, recognizing surgical pathological entities, and advancing the treatment of surgical diseases. Therefore, a large surgical revolution was being created at the time of Leeuwenhoek's discoveries.

That Leeuwenhoek did not establish a correlation between "strange little animals" and surgical disease, or disease in general, is true. That Leeuwenhoek did not presume to influence the outcome of any medical or surgical field is also true. However, that Leeuwenhoek's advances laid the foundation of upcoming surgical developments should be considered true as well.

The citizens of Delft, or the scientific world of the 17th century, cannot and should not be expected to have had the vision to accept the great discoveries of the Dutch microscopist as the early vestiges of a surgical revolution. It is more realistic to believe that Leeuwenhoek laid the first solid stones of what would be a firm and tall surgical edifice. Nearly two centuries later Louis Pasteur (1822–1895) first accepted germs as the cause of disease, and thereafter Joseph Lister (1827–1912) applied the germ theory of disease to the care of the surgical patient. In retrospect, one sees the importance of Leeuwenhoek's discoveries and that is why I consider his revolution to be a significant surgical revolution, a revolution not completely expressed until more than 100 years afterwards. Later, in other future writings, we will attach other surgical revolutions individually to Pasteur and Lister, as their contributions are equally worthy of examination.

Conclusions

Leeuwenhoek was a Dutch merchant draper and glass grinder, not a scientist, who began a series of microscopic discoveries that culminated in the identification of "strange little animals." These findings, from my own perspective, were the beginning of what should be considered a true, although delayed, surgical revolution. The details and specific reasons for his discoveries are presented within the text of this manuscript and will not be repeated in this section.

References

1. De Kruif P. (1926, reissued 1954) *Microbe Hunters.* Harvest/Harcourt Brace Jovanovich Publishers, San Diego.
2. Dobell C. (1932, reissued 1960) *Antony van Leeuwenhoek and His "Little Animals."* Russell & Russell, NY.
3. http://www.pbs.org/wnet/redgold/innovators/bio_leeuwenhoek.html. Accessed on September 17, 2008.
4. http://inventors.about.com/library/inventors/blleeuwenhoek.htm. Accessed on September 17, 2008.
5. http://www.bbc.co.uk/history/leeuwenhoek. Accessed on September 17, 2008.
6. http://www.ucmp.berkeley.edu/history/leeuwenhoek.html. Accessed on September 17, 2008.
7. Wikipedia.org/Antonie Leeuwenhoek.
8. Toledo-Pereyra LH. (2008) Surgical revolutions. *J Invest Surg* **21**:165–168.

5

Anesthesia Surgical Revolution

by Luis H. Toledo-Pereyra, MD, PhD

The discovery and use of ether for general anesthesia for surgery was an American contribution to medicine and undoubtedly the greatest development of 19th century American medicine.[1-17] Morton, Wells, Jackson, and Long were the primary players of this extraordinary tale. John Collins Warren (1778–1856), the chief surgeon at the Massachusetts General Hospital in Boston, used ether for the first time in 1846, under Morton's direction; Wells mitigated pain with nitrous oxide in his dental office in Hartford, Vermont; and Long had utilized ether in his hometown of Athens, Georgia. All of them were great contributors who fostered the development of ether for surgical anesthesia. This discovery should be considered a notable surgical revolution. To tell the saga of the American conquest of pain is not an easy undertaking since multiple players, quarrels and disagreements originated from this unique discovery. Here we give a historical description of the management of pain in general and discuss how the United States made its special mark on the medicine of the world.

Brief History of Pain Control

The history of pain relief can be traced back to ancient times. A variety of substances have been used throughout the years to dissipate pain. The Greek physician Dioscorides gave mandrake to comfort his patients.

39

Mandrake is a plant potion that induces sleep. Dioscorides claimed that mandrake produced "anesthesia," the Greek word for "without feeling." This would later become the term for the loss of sensation with or without consciousness. Chinese and Indian physicians used marijuana and hashish. Opium was also widely used in various parts of the world, as was alcohol. Willow bark, which contains salicylic acid, was at times used to decrease pain. Traveling quacks knew the value of distracting a patient's mind when undergoing surgery. This led to experimenting with hypnotism and mesmerism. In his book *We have Conquered Pain*, Dennis Fradin[9] states:

> "Surgeons were known to enter the operating room with a bottle
> of whiskey in each hand — one for the patient and the other for
> the doctor so that he could endure his patient's screams."

Prior to the emergence of ether, horror stories existed of patients screaming helplessly in pain as doctors did their work. Most patients were reluctant to undergo surgery out of fear of suffering. The main tools of a surgeon in the early 1800s were a scalpel, a bone saw, boiling water, gauze, forceps and a cauterizing iron.

Many steps were necessary before anesthesia could exist as it is known today. In 1275, Raymundus Lullius, a Spanish physician, while experimenting with chemicals, made a volatile and flammable liquid he called sweet vitriol. In 1540, a German scientist wrote of the synthesis of ether. Also in the 16th century, Paracelsus, a Swiss born physician and alchemist, made chickens breathe sweet vitriol and noted that they not only fell asleep but also felt no pain. Neither of the men ever experimented on humans. The inhalation of vapors was employed to treat a variety of aliments including phthisis, catarrh, asthma, and ureteral colic. Yet all of these elements were never considered for the treatment of human pain. In 1730, Frobenius gave sweet vitriol its present name ether, which is Greek for "heavenly."

Other Chemical Advances

In 1772, Joseph Priestley, an English scientist, discovered the gas nitrous oxide. Sir Humphrey Davy discovered the anesthetic properties of nitrous oxide. In 1800 he published *Researches, Chemical and Philosophical, chiefly concerning nitrous oxide*. In this essay, he suggested the possibilities of using nitrous oxide during surgery, based on his painless removal of a wisdom tooth. In a later publication he wrote that nitrous oxide,

> "appears capable of destroying physical pain, it may probably be used with advantage during surgical operations in which no great infusion of blood takes place."[9]

His suggestions fell on deaf ears. He was also the man who dubbed the substance "laughing gas," as an acknowledgement of the euphoria nitrous oxide induces. His student, Michael Faraday, also experimented with nitrous oxide and suggested surgical implications as well.

In 1794, English physicians Thomas Beddoes and Richard Pearson used ether to treat various ailments, including fevers and scurvy, at the Beddoes Pneumatic Institute. In 1805 American physicians used ether to treat pulmonary inflammation.

In the 1820's Henry Hickman, who was also an Englishman, conducted several experiments with anesthesia. A medical practitioner and a surgeon, he showed experimentally that carbon dioxide could induce asphyxial narcosis. Hickman sent his work to the Royal Society of London, whose president was none other than Humphrey Davy. The Royal Society was not receptive to Hickman's findings and disregarded him. This was a fortunate event since carbon dioxide was not the correct agent and, in fact, would have been very harmful.

Samuel Guthrie (1782–1848) was an American chemist, physician, and farmer. He studied medicine with his father and thereafter attended two courses, one at the College of Physicians and Surgeons in New York in 1810, and the other at the University of Pennsylvania in 1815. He then settled in New York where he produced choleric ether or chloroform in his chemical laboratories. Shortly thereafter it was discovered in Germany and France. In January 1842, William E. Clark administered ether to a patient while Dr. Elijah Pope, a dentist, extracted a tooth. The act was not publicized and was therefore not acknowledged as significant.

History of Anesthesia — Early Encounters
in the United States

The history of anesthesia is a rather complicated one since there was no clear-cut discoverer. Several individuals claimed to be the leading pioneer in the introduction of surgical anesthesia. The introduction of anesthesia was the first great medical discovery in the United States. By the mid-19th century, the world was ready for the introduction of anesthesia. The proper technology was available, and there was significant demand. Both a climate of humanitarianism and the incentive for fame and wealth steered this invention. The ignorance of the physician, due in good part to his medical education, was a reason why anesthetics were not employed at the beginning of the 19th century. When speaking of anesthesia in the 19th century, ether was administered using the "rag and bottle" technique. This consisted of placing a piece of gauze over the patient's nose and mouth and allowing drops of liquid ether or chloroform to drip onto the gauze and evaporate into a mixture of gas and air, which the patient inhaled.

Owsei Temkin, noted medical historian, has written, "Sociologists of science have cited in evidence for social causation the multiple appearance of the same discovery, 'multiples' in the language of Robert Mergon." The lack of a systematic effort to discover a method to alleviate pain may be explained by the fact that medical research at this time was based on autopsies, where pain is nonexistent. As science and society progressed, the stage was set for the introduction of anesthesia. The demonstration of ether in 1846 led Ulrich Trohler to write, "It can be seen as a heroic landmark in the history of modern surgery."[1,8,9]

The work of many scientists and physicians prepared science and medicine for the introduction of anesthesia. By most historical accounts, four major contributors (Long, Morton, Wells, and Jackson) are usually credited with the introduction of anesthesia. These four men helped bring the method into public use.

The first of the contenders for "the father of anesthesia" was Crawford Long (1815–1878), a country doctor in Danielville, Georgia. He studied at Franklin College, which would later become the University of Georgia. He received his medical training at both Transylvania University and the University of Pennsylvania in 1839. While attending medical school, Long engaged in laughing gas parties, also known as nitrous and ether frolics, which were extremely popular. At the parties nitrous oxide and ether were used as forms of entertainment. "Chemical lecturers" traveled from town to town, giving nitrous oxide demonstrations at fairs and meeting halls. When Long returned to Georgia to practice medicine, he introduced laughing gas parties to the people of his hometown. On one occasion at a laughing gas party, Long offered his friends sulfuric ether as a substitute for nitrous oxide. Long observed as a friend injured his leg without reaction while under the influence of ether. The friend acknowledged that pain existed only after his euphoria from ether had subsided.

Long recognized the medical implications of this discovery immediately. On March 30, 1842, in Jefferson, Georgia, Long successfully administered ether to James Venable, a medical student, while removing a tumor from his neck. This is the first known use of anesthesia. Two months later Long used ether while removing another tumor from the neck of the same patient. In July 1842, Long painlessly amputated a young boy's toe using ether. Within the next three years, Long successfully used ether on three more patients.

Without a doubt, Long was the first physician to use ether on patients during surgery. The reason why Long is not acclaimed as the discoverer of anesthesia is simple; he neglected to report his findings to the medical community until 1849. He published "An Account of the First Use of Sulfuric Ether by Inhalation as an Anesthetic in Surgical Operations" in the *Southern Medical and Surgical Journal* in 1849. He did, however, obtain affidavits of the efficacy of ether. At the time of his publication there were already other contenders for the title and rewards that accordingly come with being the discoverer of anesthesia.

One of these contenders was Horace Wells (1815–1848) from Hartford, Vermont. Wells was one of the leading dentists in Hartford during his time. In 1844, Wells saw a demonstration of the usefulness of ether by the popular lecturer Gardner Q. Colton (1814–1898), a disciple of P.T. Barnum. During this lecture Samuel Cooley, a participant under the influence of ether, injured his leg and did not feel any pain. This mesmerized audience members, including Horrace Wells. The experience was very similar to that of Crawford Long. Within a short period of time Wells had resolved to determine what the implications of ether would be on dentistry.

In 1844, with the aid of Dr. John M. Riggs, Wells painlessly extracted one of his own teeth. "A new era in tooth pulling," he is said to have proclaimed. What separates Wells from Long is that Wells was determined to share his discovery with the rest of the world. In January 1845, with the aid of former dentistry partner William Morton, Wells administered nitrous oxide to a patient before a medical class at Massachusetts General Hospital. This demonstration was set up by one of Boston's leading physicians and medical professors at Harvard, Dr. John C. Warren. Everything in the demonstration went according to plan until the patient unexpectedly yelled out in pain. This caused the class of medical students to boo, and the experiment was determined to be a failure. However, the patient later said that he felt no pain and had no control over his outburst. Regardless of this admission, Wells was utterly embarrassed and returned to Hartford mortified.

The third and most important contender was William Thomas Green Morton (1819–1868). Morton had dreamed of becoming a physician but did not have the financial means to achieve this goal. Instead, he was tutored by Horace Wells in dentistry in the early 1840's, and for a time in 1843 the two shared a short-lived dental practice. He also practiced dentistry in Charlestown and Boston, Massachusetts. Morton participated in the failed anesthetic demonstration by Wells. Morton claimed to have graduated from the Baltimore College of Dental Surgery; however, research has shown that he never attended medical or dental school. Nevertheless, in 1852 Washington University in Baltimore gave Morton an honorary medical degree. Morton recognized the amount of pain that existed for patients in his dental practice and began to experiment with different ways to alleviate this pain. He met with Charles Jackson, professor of chemistry and geology at Harvard and the final contender, who suggested that Morton should apply sulfuric ether to the gums of his patients. Morton began working with ether in secret, building on the principles that Jackson had taught him. He experimented with small animals at his estate in West Dedham, Massachusetts. This culminated when Morton administered ether on himself and went into an exhilarated state. At this stage Morton was prepared to make public his findings.

Using the same forum as Horace Wells, Morton planned a demonstration with the approval and support of John Collins Warren, chief surgeon at Massachusetts General. In the days and, better yet, the hours before the demonstration, Joseph M. Wightman and Nathan B. Chamberlain developed a device to administer ether. Morton and Augustus A. Gould, MD, a physician at the Massachusetts General Hospital improved upon their device. The final product was a sponge, soaked in ether, within a glass container with valves to control the dosage. On October 16, 1836 Morton successfully administered ether as Dr. Warren removed a tumor from the neck of Edward Gilbert Abbot, a man who had come to the Massachusetts General Hospital for the treatment of a vascular tumor on his jaw. This was the first victorious public administration of anesthesia. After the operation, Abbot, replying to questions about whether the procedure had hurt, stated, "No. It didn't hurt at all, although my neck did feel for a minute as if someone were scraping it with a hoe." Dr Warren is noted to have said, "Gentlemen this is no humbug," and with these words a new era in medicine began. The dome of the Bulfinch Building where the act took place was to become known as the "Ether Dome." In recent years, the administrative staff of the hospital has celebrated Ether Day every year in October to commemorate the introduction of ether to surgical anesthesia.

The Morton/Warren demonstration went so well that the very next day the duo put on another exhibition. Word quickly spread of the incredible feat, and Morton became quite famous in Boston. Dr. Oliver Wendell Holmes, the acclaimed physician-poet in Boston, knew of the Greek physician Dioscorides who had utilized the word anesthesia and recommended the name of anesthesia and anesthetics to Morton. Describing the excitement of the time the *People's Journal of London* stated,[9]

> "Oh what delight for every feeling heart to find the new year ushered in with the announcement of this noble discovery of the power to still the sense of pain, and veil the eye and memory from all the horrors of an operation...we have conquered pain."

On November 18, 1846, Dr. Henry J. Bigelow published "Insensibility During Surgical Operations Produced by Inhalation" in the *Boston Medical and Surgical Journal.* The article recounted how Bigelow had witnessed four operations in the previous months, in which Morton administered anesthesia while Dr. John Collins Warren or Dr. George Hayward performed the procedure. This article quickly excited the medical community in Boston, and they gave Morton all of the backing for discovering anesthesia. In 1847, Morton published "Proper Mode of Administering Sulfuric Ether by Inhalation" in an attempt to promote his work. Before describing the events following Morton's demonstration the final actor should be discussed.

Charles Jackson (1805–1880) called Plymouth, Massachusetts, his home. Jackson spent much of his time dabbling in science, especially chemistry, physiology, and geology. He was also an unknown inventor, a professor at Harvard, and a noted tutor. In 1844, Jackson argued that he had suggested using ether to soothe patients' pain to William Morton. This is Jackson's primary claim to being the founder of anesthesia. Jackson proposed that he was unknowingly aiding a friend, who then used his knowledge and insight against him. Jackson asserted that he was the true discoverer of the benefits of ether and that Morton simply stole what was rightfully his. At the same time that Morton was giving lectures in Boston about the implications of his discovery, Jackson was doing the same. However, Jackson's audiences were less receptive to his claims.

Following the use of ether, chloroform became the anesthetic of choice. James Y. Simpson, head of obstetrics at Edinburg, first introduced chloroform to relieve obstetrical pain in Scotland in 1847. Ether was known to have a bad odor, irritated the lungs, made patients vomit, and required awkward equipment. This led directly to the more frequent use of chloroform, which was quicker, cheaper, more powerful and lasted longer. It should be noted however, that excessive amounts of either chloroform or ether were known to produce serious side effects and even death.

Difficulties in Assigning a Single Discoverer

After the various incidents, these pioneering men engaged in a bitter battle of who was the true discoverer of anesthesia. For different reasons, all men had a partial claim. The controversy spread all the way to Congress, the newspapers, and Europe. Morton, in an attempt to make a profit, created a substance called Letheon by simply adding oil of citrus to mask the telltale odor of ether. Adding to the controversy was that the United States granted William Morton a patent, U.S. patent #4848 on November 12, 1846, for his method of etherization, which used a glass jar with a rubber tube. Morton gave up his dental practice to concentrate on promoting Letheon, causing him great economic hardship. Contributing to Morton's state of financial plight was the fact that even the U.S. government would not pay him royalties on his patent. This was demonstrated during the Mexican-American War (1846–1848) when the army used its own inhaling devices without paying Morton a cent. This, in effect, sent a message to surgeons and dentists that it was not necessary to recognize Morton's patent. Several times Congress came close to allocating $100,000 as a reward to Morton. However, the appropriations bill never passed the Senate. When it eventually became clear that Congress was not going to award any of the men any monetary prize for their discoveries, then-President Franklin Pierce urged Morton to sue the U.S. government for $100,000 for its employment of etherization during the Mexican-American War. It was Pierce's belief that this was the only manner in which Morton could be compensated for his efforts. The case remained in the court system until 1862, when the decision was rendered that Morton would receive nothing since what he had patented was a procedure and therefore was unpatentable, a nonsensical attitude in light of the patent law of today.

Results of the Battle for Supremacy

The battle over credit for discovering the use of ether was not without casualties. Jackson made several attempts to claim priority both in the United States and France. With unconvincing evidence and a less-than-credible history, Jackson met very little success in his campaign. He had earlier sued Samuel Morse over the invention of the telegraph. He also claimed to have invented guncotton, an explosive. Jackson eventually was committed to a mental asylum, where he remained until his death. It is said that Jackson went mad upon reading Morton's tombstone, which acknowledged Morton as the inventor of inhaled anesthesia.

Horace Wells also attempted to claim priority in Washington, with little fruition. Like Jackson, Wells' life turned tragic in his attempt to earn credit for his role in discovering anesthesia. Wells privately continued experimenting with forms of anesthesia and soon became addicted to chloroform. In 1848 he was arrested for throwing acid on a prostitute, while under the influence of the drug. Two days later while in prison, Wells committed suicide by severing his femoral artery.

Morton, on account of the priority dispute, was rendered penniless and was constantly on the verge of a nervous breakdown. This is well reviewed by James Thomas Flexner in *The Death of Pain*, which hailed Long as Morton's co-discoverer. Morton died of a stroke in 1868, never achieving the widespread acclaim that he so sought. His headstone does bear a legacy in the inscription by Dr. Jacob Bigelow,

> "Inventor, Revealer of Anaesthetic Inhalation. By whom pain in surgery was averted and annulled. Before whom in all time surgery was agony. Since whom science has control of pain."

Long was the only one of the four men to live to see old age. He remained a country physician until his death. Long, in contrast to the others, lived a happy, honest, and decent life. Fittingly, he had never sought to profit from his discoveries. In the south, Long did have many supporters, who proposed that he was the first to introduce surgical etherization.

Final Outcome and Consequences

In general, the use of anesthesia was quickly accepted in most sectors of society. Before the end of 1846, ether was administered during surgical procedures in both Paris and London. In England, in December 1846, Robert Liston successfully amputated a limb, pain-free. However, it was not a smooth and seamless road to the anesthesia of today. For instance, a noted Philadelphia surgeon, H.H. Smith commented in 1852 that "I have myself affected by extreme lassitude from breathing the atmosphere...during a prolonged etherization." The clergy initially opposed the use of anesthesia, believing that it contradicted God's plan for mankind's suffering. This was especially the case when used during childbirth. The Church believed that misery in childbirth was God's punishment for Eve's transgression in the Garden. On the other hand, Morton commented "unrestrained and free as God's own sunshine, ether has gone forth to cheer and gladden the earth' it will awaken the gratitude of the present, and all coming generations." However, Morton's comments regarding the public's reaction should not be viewed without bias, given his self-promoting behavior.

John Snow was the first professional anesthetist in Great Britain. He worked at St. George's Hospital in Hyde Park Corner, London. In 1847 he invented a portable ether inhaler. The first known instance of ether being applied during childbirth was to Fannie Appleton Longfellow in 1847. Also in 1847, Walter Channing, Dean of the Medical School at Harvard, published a work on *Etherization and Childbirth*, hailing the possibilities of the resent discovery. In 1853, Queen Victoria used chloroform during the birth of her eighth child, Prince Leopold, thereby making it an acceptable practice. This royal validation came at an important point, as not everyone was fully convinced of the great benefits of anesthesia.

Pierre Flourens, a 19th century philosopher, argued that "with the increasing superficiality of the general training of our doctors, the unlimited use of chloroform may encourage surgeons to carry out complex and difficult operations." This helped to further the argument that the new anesthetic procedure could help patients who otherwise did not have an opportunity to be treated for diseases that might require extensive surgery. Flourens did have a valid point; surgeons were encouraged to perform more complex operations and thereby advanced medical science.

There is a widely held misconception that soldiers were never given anesthesia during the Civil War. This is not the case. By the 1860s opposition to anesthesia was rare in the United States. In 1862, a lecturer at the College of Physicians and Surgeons in New York asserted that "the day is past where the administration of anesthetics in surgical operations is subject for discussion." The benefits that ether and chloroform produced quickly hushed their opponents in the medical debate over their use. Professor J.J. Chisolm summarized the attitude of Confederate surgeons in his *Manual of Military Surgery*:[3]

> "The universal use of chloroform to allay the pain of surgical operations is a complete vindication for the utility of this remedy, and proof of its necessity...We do not hesitate to say that it should be given to every patient requiring a serious or painful operation."

During the course of the war, Union records showed that at least 80,000 operations were done using anesthesia and only 254 were completed without. Clearly, the use of anesthetics was an accepted practice.

During the Civil War, the pioneers of anesthesia were serving in various military capacities. Morton served as a volunteer battlefield anesthetist for the Union. He eventually attended more than 2,000 soldiers. He took an average of three minutes to administer anesthesia to a fallen soldier on the battlefield. On the opposing side, Long was in charge of the Confederate hospital in Athens, Georgia. Long had the foresight to order enormous amounts of ether and chloroform, which proved instrumental in the many operations that he performed during the war. By this time, in the mid-1860's, chloroform was the most frequent general anesthetic used (in an approximate scale of five to one compared to ether).

In spite of the overwhelming use of anesthetics by the time of the war, it was not until the 1870's that anesthesia was a constant fixture in the medical arena. This lack of complete acceptance occurred for several reasons. Many doctors thought that the use of anesthesia brought the patient too close to death. It was also a widespread belief that pain was a necessary part of the healing process. Some physicians believed that the use of ether or chloroform was not natural, which fed off the popular appeal of irregulars and homeopaths.

The debate over who should receive credit for the introduction of anesthesia was never truly resolved. In 1864, the American Dental Association deemed Wells as the discoverer of anesthesia, and in 1870, the American Medical Association followed suit. In 1877, Dr. J. Marion Sims published "The Discovery of Anesthesia" in the *Virginia Medical Monthly* journal. It was the first work to acknowledge that all four men had together substantially contributed to the discovery of anesthesia. Perhaps this is the most accurate account. Crawford Long was the first to use a new process. Horace Wells was the first to advocate widespread use in a populous area and made Boston more receptive for William Morton, who made anesthesia an accepted part of medicine. Finally, it is undeniable that Charles Jackson's suggestions were vital to Morton's success.

What has been the Impact of the Introduction of Anesthesia?

Today people have the opportunity to receive painless surgery. With the emerging acceptance of the germ theory of disease and ensuing antiseptic and aseptic methods developed in the 1870's, more complex surgeries would become possible. John Galbraith Simmons describes the climate of the time best:[15]

> "Surgery reinvented itself in the late 19th century. While advances in physiology and pathology made it possible to understand the architecture and some of the dynamics of the human body, anesthesia and asepsis made it plausible to open it up and repair it."

It took many decades for anesthetics to advance to what is now known in the 21st century. Even into the early 1900's, the specialty of anesthesia still consisted of dropping ether via a soaked sponge into a patient's nose. Little attention was given to vital signs during the operative procedure until 1895 when Harvey Cushing noticed the high rates of ether overdose. After blaming himself for the death of a patient due to excessive anesthesia, Cushing and an associate developed the anesthesia record or "ether charts." Following his initiative, blood pressure, pulse, and respiratory rate began to be monitored.

By the end of the first half of the 20th century, the profession of anesthesiology required four to five years of graduate education after medical school. Today, because of the immeasurable benefits of anesthesia, each year in the U.S. alone, millions of surgeries are being performed with the administration of anesthesia. By itself, this discovery represents a unique surgical revolution. There is no question that because of the discovery of anesthesia, society now has the benefit of medical and dental procedures without fear of pain, a luxury that generations past never dreamed possible.

References

1. *Agony!: From Agony to Anesthesia*. JLR Medical Group. (2002) Available at: http://www.jlrmedicalgroup.com/agony.htm.
2. Angle G, Harding RS, Crawford W. *Long Collection, 1842–1926, #120.* Available at http://americanhistory.si.edu/archives/d9120/htm.
3. Bollet AJ. (2002) *Civil War Medicine: Challenges and Triumphs.* Galen Press, Ltd., Tucson, AZ.
4. Clarke E. (1971) *Modern Methods in the History of Medicine.* Athlone Press of the University of London, London.

5. Doyle SR. *Anesthetic Agents: Inhaled Anesthetics.* October 18, 2000. Available at: http://www.nurse-anesthesia.com/inhaledanesthetics.htm.

6. Duffy J. (1993) *From Humors to Medical Science.* Second Edition. University of Illinois, Champaign, IL.

7. Evans T. The Unusual History of Ether. *Anesthesia Nursing and Medicine.* (2003) Available at http://www.anesthesia-nursing.com/ether.html.

8. Fenster JM. (2001) *Ether Day.* Perennial Harper Collins, New York.

9. Fradin DB. (1996) *We have Conquered Pain: the Discovery of Anesthesia.* Margaret K. McElderry Books, New York.

10. Friedman G, Friedman M. (1998) *Medicine's 10 Greatest Discoveries.* Yale University Press, New Haven, CT.

11. Gordon R. (1993) *The Alarming History of Pain: Amusing Anecdotes from Hippocrates to Heart Transplants.* St. Martin's Press, New York.

12. History of Anesthesia. *Anesthesia Today.* (1999) Available at: http://204.178.120.164/history.asp.

13. *Medicine's Greatest Gift.* Neurosurgical Service, Massachusetts General Hospital and Harvard University. (2000) Available at: http://neurosurgery.mgh.harvard.edu/History/gift.htm.

14. Nuland SB. (1983) *The Origins of Anesthesia.* The Classics of Medicine Library, Birmingham, AL.

15. Simmons JG. (2002) *Doctors and Discoveries: Lives That Created Today's Medicine, from Hippocrates to the Present.* Houghton Mifflin Company, Boston.

16. Toledo-Pereyra LH. (2005) *Vignettes On Surgery, History and Humanities.* Landes Bioscience, Georgetown, TX.

17. Vertosick FT. (2000) *Why We Hurt: The Natural History Of Pain.* Harcourt Inc., Sherman Oaks, CA.

Introduction A L'Etude de la Medicine Experimentale Surgical Revolution, Part I

by Luis H. Toledo-Pereyra, MD, PhD

No other book in 19th century medicine was more influential than the *Introduction a L'Etude de la Medicine Experimentale* written by Claude Bernard (1813–1878) and successfully published in France in 1865.[1-11] All scientists worldwide greatly admired this unique book of philosophical scientific inquiry. Its influence extended far beyond medicine into the confines of surgery, which is why I am discussing the book here.

Brief Biographical Details

Claude Bernard originated from Saint-Julien, France, where he was born on July 12, 1813.[9] He received his early education nearby, with strong Catholic emphasis particularly from his mother and the parish priest.[9] He attended college at Lyon and worked for an apothecary before moving to Paris in 1834 to pursue a career in literature.[9] Little did he know that medicine and physiology were to be his future.

Apparently discouraged by a literary critic, Bernard left behind his literary ambitions and moved into medicine. After barely passing his

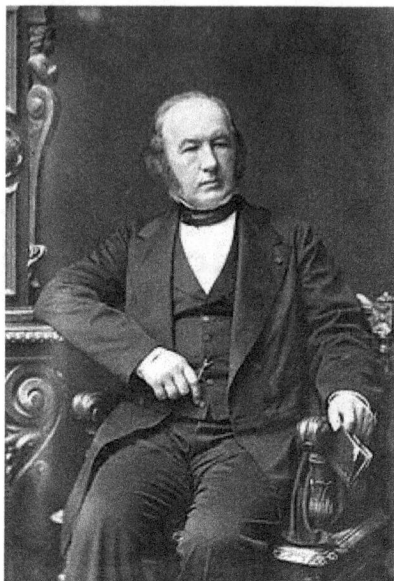

Figure 6.1.   Photograph of Bernard in later life. No date or source identified.

baccalaureate, he gained admission to the Faculty of Medicine in Paris. His biographers considered Bernard as an average student without showing a brilliant mind.[9] However, no one predicted his extraordinary ascent to the prestigious Academic Francaise.

In 1839, he passed his examinations for internship at Paris Municipal Hospitals. Under these circumstances, he worked on the staff of Francois Magendie at Hotel Dieu. Magendie's personality and bold approach to science, combined with intense skepticism, greatly impressed Bernard's young mind. In Magendie's laboratory Bernard found his new life as an experimental physiologist,[9] a life which would become the pride of France, the pride of the world of physiology, and the pride of medical and surgical advances.

In 1841, Bernard officially became the *preparateur* to Magendie at the College de France. In this position, he assisted the professor in various kinds of experiments, such as exploring the physiology of the spinal nerve roots, the cerebrospinal fluid, the origin of oxidation in horses, and the physiology of digestion.[4,5,9] The use of animal vivisection constituted an essential part of Magendie's research, and obviously Bernard learned each

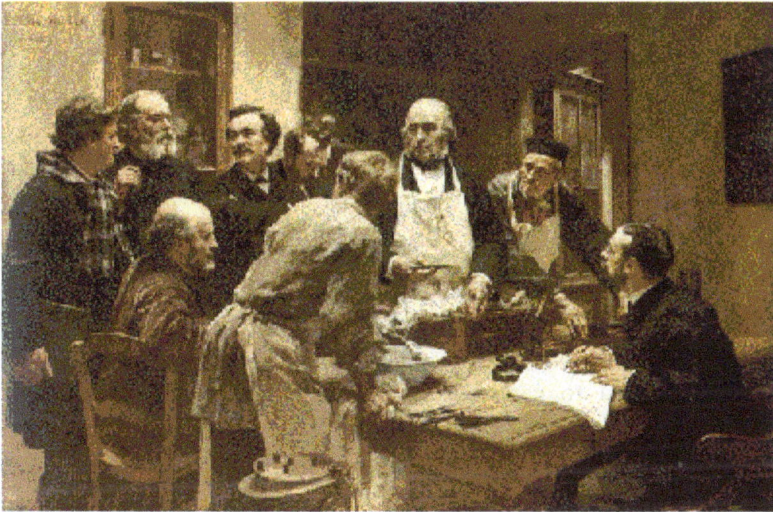

Figure 6.2. The Lesson of Claude Bernard (1889). Oil painting by Leon-Agustin L'hermitte (1844–1915). This is an artistic depiction of animal vivisection at the College of France. Currently maintained at the Paris Academy of Medicine.

one of the details associated with it, particularly in regards to advancing medical research. Bernard followed his master's principles very closely, even though skepticism and empiricism were not an important part of Bernard's thinking and philosophical approach.

In 1843, Bernard obtained his medical doctor degree with an impressive medical thesis examining new concepts of gastric digestion and its role in nutrition.[4,6,9] By this time, Bernard's interest in research was established, and he never practiced clinical medicine during his professional life. He remained a committed physiologist and experimentalist throughout his prolific and notable career.

A year later, in 1844, Bernard could not pass the examinations for securing a teaching position at the Faculty of Medicine, but this negative event only temporarily detracted from his ultimate goals of research and teaching. However, it took three years before he would be reincorporated into Parisian academia. Meanwhile, he finished his laboratory position with Magendie and married Fanny Martin in 1845, daughter of a Paris doctor whose finances allowed him to continue his personal physiological research.[9]

In 1847, the Saint-Julien future master returned to Magendie Laboratories at the College de France in full force. He accepted a position as Magendie's deputy-professor and began the most significant period of his outstanding scientific career. In 1852, Magendie retired as expected and his favorite student followed as the most deserving physiologist to occupy his notable chair.[5,9] Few medical scientists in France were more qualified than the advanced student to take over his master's distinguished job.

In 1853, Bernard obtained a doctorate in zoology from the Sorbonne with special emphasis on new functions of the liver and, in particular, related to carbohydrate metabolism, which would culminate in discoveries pertaining to animal glycogenesis.[9] Bernard continued his active research and commitment to teaching in the following years until early 1860, when his health began to fail for variable periods of time.[9]

As the 1860's began to unfold, Bernard dedicated more time to the integration of research methods and the development of philosophical principles in research, medicine and science. The positivism of Comte became a source of interest for Bernard, even though critical in nature.[9] The philosophy of the accomplished physiologist was complex but clear, one in which determinism was emphasized.

In the 1870's, between periods of good health, Bernard assumed his teaching periodically. His research was less frequent. By the end of the decade, Bernard's health was in continuous decay and in 1878 he died, probably of kidney failure.[9] A national funeral followed, which is not a surprise in the case of Bernard.

Bernard the Scientist

Bernard dedicated his productive professional life to the study of scientific phenomena. Understanding their nature, delving into their causes, and advancing laboratory hypotheses were the main concerns of the innovative French physiologist. His studies were clear, well-organized and followed research principles we still use today. In many ways, Bernard outlined the basis for the research being conducted in our time.

The research work of Bernard was extensive and it is not our intention to cover all his well-designed and successful studies.[9] By way of summary, it would be important to recognize certain areas of his extraordinary science. First, the glycogenic function of the liver, which shed light on the way that glucose is metabolized in the liver, is probably his more identifiable discovery.[4,10] Second, the function of the pancreatic juice as a substantial element in the digestive process presented Bernard as an advanced and thoughtful researcher. Third, the characterization and discovery of the vasomotor nervous system placed Bernard at the top of the physiological world, since in addition to his previous findings he could readily discern the effect of vasodilator and vasoconstrictor nerves.

Bernard opened the new doors of modern physiology, which made him the father of modern experimental physiology.[5,9] Many more discoveries came from Bernard; the list is long and worth reviewing through some of his original publications as extensively presented by M.D. Grmek,[9] one of the distinguished students of Bernard's life and accomplishments.

As principled and dedicated a researcher as Bernard was, he could not solve all the physiological and experimental problems in medicine being considered at that point in time. Bernard was an excellent experimentalist and superb researcher but did not have all the answers for all the questions presented to him. What Bernard had, however, was a firm desire to resolve all vexing and critical areas in the medicine of his day.

Bernard brought with him an innovative mind, a special intellect and a determination in research to advance to levels not reached in the medicine or surgery of his times. It was evident that this accomplished French researcher had a firm path oriented at identifying the complicated issues of medical sciences.

Bernard learned his first research ideas and methods for testing them from his master Magendie. And, even though his personality had much to be desired, Bernard was able to obtain the best he could from the good side of his teacher. Bernard was in constant pursuit of answers for his research projects; he was drawn by the experimental method and its application. Bernard was a true experimentalist and a true believer in the scientific method. He believed in supporting his ideas with well sought-out facts. Bernard was the consummate researcher.

Scientific Determinism

Bernard understood better than any other scientist of his time the value of pure science. Bernard was a physician who never practiced medicine and entirely dedicated himself to the delights of the scientific process. Bernard believed in *scientific determinism*, which could be summarized in one sentence: "Identical experiments have identical results."[5]

Some practitioners of medicine and surgery and basic scientists did not support the principle of *scientific determinism* introduced by Bernard. A few were in favor of *vitalism*, which represented a "vital force" behaving in an "arbitrary and unpredictable way."[5] Others did not follow a particular school of thought. A few more considered that science did not follow determinism or vitalism specifically, but a combination of the two. Many more, however, were in favor of Bernard's beliefs of *scientific determinism*.

It is important to clarify, that in 1847 according to Tarshis,[5] only a few individuals were involved in science. France, Germany and England, the leading European nations, had few medical scientists working in laboratories doing basic research. France, the leader in medical sciences during the first part of the 19th century, had practically no one working on experimental medicine, except for Magendie initially and later on Bernard, who opened this field for all to try!

In the French Parisian medical schools or centers of medical learning of the day, experimental medicine was rarely considered or its presence was infrequently accepted. Physicians and surgeons, in general, accepted practical concepts but not the theoretical dilemmas brought in from the halls of basic sciences. Skepticism reigned over all the confines of the clinical wards and the elementary boundaries of the operating rooms. Bernard was convinced that medicine and science were joined together and could not be readily separated. Based on his principles of *scientific determinism*, Bernard was committed to answering many of the quandaries existing with the medicine of the day. "Bernard insisted that the study of disease must not be separate from the study of health since there is only one science of life."[5]

Millieu Interieur

Bernard, among many significant developments, created the term *milieu interieur* to explain how the internal environment would give us a balanced and stable condition within the normal function of the human body. This would be compared later on to the homeostasis principle introduced by the noted American physiologist, Walter Cannon.

Bernard believed that disease was caused, in great part, by a "faulty regulation of the internal environment."[5] This concept was definitely ahead of his times and was not understood when he introduced it in one of his magisterial lectures given on December 17, 1875.[5] According to Tarshis, Bernard came out gradually with this concept of internal environment.[5] Initially, he used it to support his idea of experimental medicine and later on to counteract the "vital force" concepts presented by the "vitalists" as a way to understand the function of the living organism.[5] For Bernard, the "vital force" was "nonsense."[5]

As time evolved, Bernard readjusted the original ideas of the *milieu interieur*, combining the functions of the external and internal environments. Let us hear Bernard in his own words[5]:

> "The fixity of the *milieu interieur* supposes a perfection of the organism such that the external variations are at each instant compensated for and equilibrated. Therefore, far from being indifferent to the external world...(an) equilibrium results from a continuous and delicate compensation established as if by the most sensitive of balances."

In short, according to Grmek[9] "the notion of 'milieu interieur' occupies a central place in Bernard's thought." From animal experiments, over time, Bernard progressed to a more sophisticated state when the "milieu" was either responsible for or the effect of a pathological state.

For Bernard, the "milieu" was "the precondition of a free, independent life."[9]

The Book — *Introduction A L'Etude de la Medicine Experimentale*

Eighteen sixty-five marked the year of publication of one of the best books, or perhaps *the* best book, written about medical scientific philosophy of the 19th century, and one could even contend that is the best book ever written on this topic.

Why is this book so important? Because Claude Bernard gave us his life and experience in medical physiological research in a matter never presented before. He was clear, frank, detailed and offered superb advice to young investigators in experimental medicine, and by logical extension to clinical researchers as well.

Bernard made numerous important observations throughout this work. His astute recommendations as to how to improve the planning, development and execution of research are well-covered. Bernard speaks as the master researcher he was. He emphasized more than anything gathering facts, since facts are the only generators of truth, scientific evidence, and medical advancement.

References

1. Bergson H. (1975) *An Introduction to Metaphysics. The Creative Mind.* Translated into English by Andison ML. Littlefield, Adams & Co., Totowa, NJ.
2. Holmes FL. (1974) *Claude Bernard and Animal Chemistry. The Emergence of a Scientist.* Harvard University Press, Cambridge, MA.
3. Virtanen R. (1960) *Claude Bernard and His Place in the History of Ideas.* University of Nebraska Press, Lincoln, Nebraska.
4. Grande F, Visscher MB (eds.). (1967) *Claude Bernard and Experimental Medicine.* Schenkman Publishing Co., Inc., Cambridge, MA.
5. Tarshis J. (1968) *Claude Bernard. Father of Experimental Medicine.* The Dial Press, Inc., New York.
6. Hoff HE. (1958) Claude Bernard's introduction. A review. *Bull Hist Med* **XXIX**:177–181.

7. Riese W. (1943) Claude Bernard on the light of modern science. *Bull Hist Med* **XIV**:281–294.

8. Normandin S. (2007) Claude Bernard. An introduction to the study of experimental medicine: "physical vitalism," dialectic and epistemology. *J Hist Med* **62**:495–528.

9. Grmek MD. (1970) Bernard, Claude. In: CC Gillespie, (ed.). *Dictionary of Scientific Biography*. Vol. II. Charles Scribner's Sons, New York, 1970, pp. 24–34.

10. Sinding C. (1999) Claude Bernard and Louis Pasteur. Contrasting images through public commemorations. *Osiris* **14**:65–81.

11. Bernard C. (1957) *An Introduction to the Study of Experimental Medicine*. Dover Publications Inc., New York.

7

Introduction A L'Etude de la Medicine Experimentale, Part II

by Luis H. Toledo-Pereyra, MD, PhD

Introduction

The book written by Claude Bernard on experimental medicine revolutionized the way that physicians and surgeons saw and interpreted the medicine of the day, as well as the medicine practiced by future generations of clinicians and clinical researchers.[1-11] In Part I of the *Introduction à l'Étude de la Médecine Expérimentale*,[12] we advanced the genius of Bernard, his life and accomplishments and his evolution as a scientist, then began evaluating the influence of his book on medicine and surgery. In Part II we continue the critical assessment of Bernard's classic book of experimental medicine and establish the reasons behind the development of a surgical revolution.

Bernard saw the experimental method as divided into three stages: observation, hypothesis and experimentation.[1-11] Experimental reasoning was at the origin of the research enterprise, according to the acclaimed French physiologist.[9] Philosophical questions of the experimental method interested Bernard a great deal. Everything had a reason and was explained through a series of well-gathered facts.

Research without proven facts did not exist in the mind of Bernard,[9,11] since facts gave research the essence of its existence. "Experimental

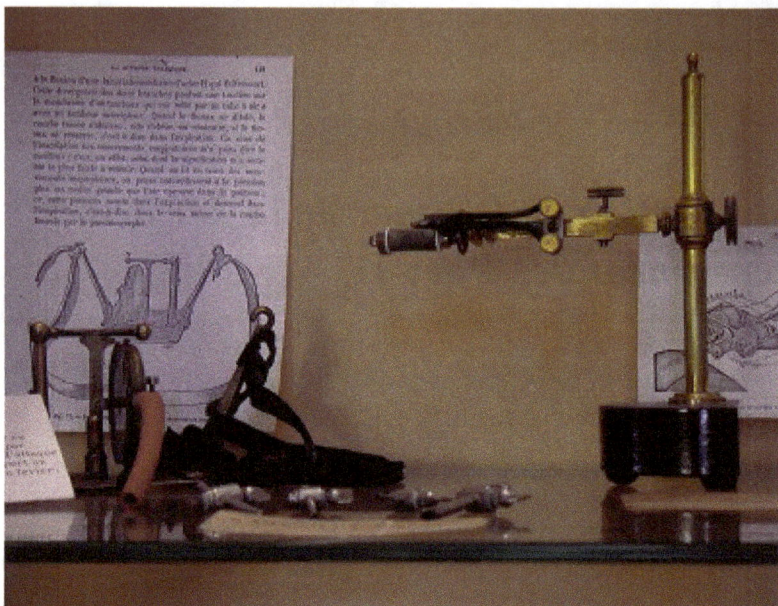

Figure 7.1.   Display of instruments used for Bernard's research.

verification" was a necessary element to confirm the hypothesis and the whole research idea.[11] Bernard was very clear about all research concepts and particularly about demonstrating the best means to gather the most accurate information. The *Introduction* was replete with these various observations and recommendations.

According to Grmek:

> "The success of the *Introduction* is due, at least in part, to the glimpse that it affords of the personal adventures of a great biologist and its claims to the revelation of the secrets of his scientific success. In fact, almost all the examples cited by Bernard in support of his general concepts stem from his own work."[9]

Without further consideration, it is credible to believe that Bernard's *Introduction* presented to the world of research and medicine something that was new, educational, informative and encouraging as far as medical research was concerned. Bernard's book had approached the philosophy of medical research in a manner that others had not written about previously. Bernard was ahead of his times and saw medical experimentation in unique and innovative ways and this made his book the best available on philosophical medical and surgical research.

Bernard on Statistics in Biology and Medicine

Determinism and averages were important to Bernard. But he cautioned regarding the excessive "use of averages," which he considered to be statistics in biology.[6,11] He was concerned about some inaccuracies of statistical methods and how the application of these principles was not always conducive to saving lives![1] Bernard gave us an example of his thinking in the *Introduction*:[11]

> "A great surgeon performs operations for stone by a single method; later he makes a statistical summary of deaths and recoveries, and he concludes from these statistics that the mortality law for this operation is two out of five. Well, I say that this ratio means literally nothing scientifically and gives us no certainty in performing the next operation; for we do not know whether the next case will be among the recoveries or the deaths. What really should be done, instead of gathering facts empirically, is to study them more accurately, each in its special determinism ... to discover in them the cause of mortal accidents so as to master the cause and avoid the accidents."

For Bernard, the statistical methods "lead to probabilities, at best they may suggest research."[11,13] Bernard walked terrain that was difficult to assess in 19th century science, particularly in 19th century medical clinical sciences.

The caution expressed by Bernard about the use of statistics is real today, since a careful conclusion should be reached only after evaluating each case individually. Even though the statistics will help in the final assessment, Bernard did not give to statistics the only and absolute value. This approach was good then and appears to be reasonable under certain circumstances today.

The Basis for a Surgical Revolution

Bernard's *Introduction* was not only important for medical research but for researchers involved in the surgical sciences as well. The importance was significant enough to constitute not only a medical revolution but also, and more evidently, a surgical revolution. Initially surgical research began with surgeons interested in answering some of their clinical problems. Later on, at the end of the 19th century, some American surgeons and their European counterparts pursued research in their medical schools' academic centers. The teachings of Bernard, well-represented by his magnificent book the *Introduction*, served as the most important source of learning for those surgeons who wanted to conduct research like the French master had. Other books by Bernard emphasizing operative surgery and surgical anatomy, published in 1856 and 1866, were favorites among many American surgeons.[4]

Even though we do not have a direct way to find which surgeons read Bernard's book individually, the manner in which they approached their research presents to us some indirect evidence that, at some point, they learned Bernard's research principles. More specifically, if one studies the research lives of master surgeons like Theodor Kocher (1841–1917), William Halsted (1852–1922) or Owen Wangensteen (1898–1981) at the beginning of the 20th century, it is not difficult to consider that they had read or learned Bernard's background and research essentials. Kocher in Europe and the two Americans, Halsted and Wangensteen, who had spent more than a year under European influence early in their careers, had in one way or another received Bernard's principles of research as expressed in the *Introduction*.

Disciples of Kocher, Halsted and Wangensteen, and disciples of their disciples, and many other American and European surgeons who were interested in surgical research, most likely had the opportunity to hear, read or be shown the research ideas presented by Bernard in his classic book.

In 1962, when I was a second year medical student in my class of physiology at the National Autonomous University of Mexico (UNAM), I was exposed for the first time by Professor Carlos Alcocer to the deeds and writings of Claude Bernard, particularly the research ideas of his book, *Introduction*. Years later, when I moved to the University of Minnesota and began my surgical research laboratory time, in 1972, under Surgeon Director Dr. John S. Najarian, I became keenly aware of Bernard's book, bought a copy and read it frequently. Just about the same time, my studies on the history of medicine, under Medical historian Dr. Leonard G. Wilson, provided me with an improved perspective of Bernard's work. I became convinced then and believe today that Bernard created — with his philosophical scientific writings — a surgical revolution to be better recognized by those involved in the surgical research sciences.

Concluding Remarks

The extraordinary book of Bernard, the *Introduction*, represented the most advanced philosophical medical research book of the time and we could add the best book of all time on its subject matter. Because of the unique contributions of Bernard's book on the conception, preparation, development and culmination of the research study, medical and surgical researchers benefited a great deal. From our own perspective, without Bernard's book, surgeon researchers would not have advanced the knowledge of surgical research at the pace observed through the years, and therefore, we propose that this book represented a surgical revolution for surgeons working in research and the clinical sciences as well.

References

1. Bergson H. (1975) *An Introduction to Metaphysics. The Creative Mind.* Translated into English by Andison ML. Littlefield, Adams & Co., Totowa, NJ.
2. Holmes FL. (1974) *Claude Bernard and Animal Chemistry. The Emergence of a Scientist.* Harvard University Press, Cambridge, MA.
3. Virtanen R. (1960) *Claude Bernard and His Place in the History of Ideas.* University of Nebraska Press, Lincoln, NE.
4. Grande F, Visscher MB (eds.). (1967) *Claude Bernard and Experimental Medicine.* Schenkman Publishing Co., Inc., Cambridge, MA.
5. Tarshis J. (1968) *Claude Bernard. Father of Experimental Medicine.* The Dial Press, Inc., New York.
6. Hoff HE. (1958) Claude Bernard's Introduction. A review. *Bull Hist Med* **XXIX**:177–181.

7. Riese W. (1943) Claude Bernard on the light of modern science. *Bull Hist Med* **XIV**:281–294.

8. Normandin S. (2007) Claude Bernard. An introduction to the study of experimental medicine: "physical vitalism," dialectic and epistemology. *J Hist Med* **62**:495–528.

9. Grmek MD. (1970) Bernard, Claude. In: CC Gillespie (ed.). *Dictionary of Scientific Biography.* Vol. II. Charles Scribner's Sons, New York.

10. Sinding C. (1999) Claude Bernard and Louis Pasteur. Contrasting images through public commemorations. *Osiris* **14**:65–81.

11. Bernard C. (1957) *An Introduction to the Study of Experimental Medicine.* Dover Publications Inc., New York.

12. Toledo-Pereyra LH. (2009) Introduction à *l'Étude de la Médecine Expérimentale.* Surgical Revolution. Part I. *J Invest Surg* **22**:157–161.

13. Bernard C. Available at http://en.wikipedia.org/wiki/claude_bernard. Accessed on May 8, 2009.

8

Joseph Lister Surgical Revolution

by Luis H. Toledo-Pereyra, MD, PhD

Joseph Lister (1827–1912), without a doubt, represented the most accomplished scientific surgeon of his time. He made contributions to the field that became the basis upon which the surgery of today relies in all its vigor and expression. Lister brought to the surgical field the understanding and appreciation of antiseptic principles, identifying the direct relationship between microorganisms and surgical disease, and this knowledge was conducive to decreasing surgical morbidity and mortality.

Lister created antiseptic surgery and, therefore, created a true surgical revolution that saved thousands of patients during the perioperative period. No other procedure or surgical discovery that had been introduced before had such a great impact on the surgical specialty as antiseptic surgery when locally or systematically applied.

Antiseptic Surgical Revolution

In March 1867, Lister claimed to have found a new method for treating compound fractures and advancing the cure of suppurations from the bone and soft tissues of patients suffering from injuries producing these fractures.[1,2] The mortality associated with these conditions was staggering. Nothing proposed before Lister had any demonstrable effect on these untreatable septic problems.

69

Lister described 11 cases with only one death, a result unheard of previously.[1-13] What was occurring was not understood. Surgeons could not believe that Lister's concepts or Listerism was the cause of it. Indeed, the surgical and medical world was completely apathetic to Lister's developments.

How, then, did Lister implement a consistent solution to the high mortality that followed the treatment of compound fractures? How did he change the paradigm of treatment for unsolved surgical or operative infections? What did he use that would modify the world's management and treatment of infected surgical wounds? What was so different in his approach and his way of understanding disease?

I believe Lister's solution to the dismal management of surgical wounds was reached based on three different fundamental factors: one, his knowledge and practice of basic sciences applicable to surgery; two, his belief in the germ theory of disease; and three, his understanding that antiseptics were needed to overcome infection. We have previously written about the fundamental conditions upon which Lister based his theory and results.[3-8] Now, the idea is to place them into perspective regarding the overall effect these monumental findings, published in 1867,[1] had on surgery then and today.

The revolutions in surgery, in any other area of medicine, or for that matter, in any particular field of scientific endeavor or humanistic approach, require a vastly different consideration. Revolution is a radical change, compatible only with a cataclysm, a new way to see things, something never seen before. And that was what the antiseptic method of Lister represented.

Lister's Reasons for the Application of the Antiseptic Method

The factors determining the manner in which Lister approached the problem of sepsis during and immediately after surgery were generated from the basic understanding he had of wound suppuration and infection after the operative act. This consideration, combined with his knowledge of Pasteur's findings on the germ theory of disease, was critical to his application of the antiseptic method in 1865 — the results of which were published in 1867.[1,2]

Lister had a clear understanding of the science behind the presence of infections in surgical wounds. The microorganisms were the evident culprits and needed to be combated. Pasteur had opened the doors and

Lister, using the French scientist's knowledge, followed a logical path to understanding how the wounds got infected. In order to think like Lister, it is necessary to think about the germ theory of disease, or to think like Pasteur, if you prefer to see it in that way.[2]

Now, how did Lister change the paradigm of unsolved surgical infections? Consider the larger equation, since believing in the germ theory would clarify the whys and why-nots of this complex and unsolved problem. Lister followed his convictions, applied his knowledge and reached the solution. Wounds were infected by microorganisms, which he needed to get rid of in order to improve a patient's condition. In hindsight, this solution appears very simple. Get rid of the infection and the patient will be fine!

What did Lister use that would modify the world's management and treatment of infected surgical wounds? As we have said before, he used his surgical principles of wound management, which were based on no germs, no infected wounds, and no disease. It is hard to understand why others had not seen these relationships before. The reason resides in the preparation and ideas of Lister, which culminated in his extraordinary results.

What was so different in Lister's approach and understanding of wound surgical disease? Quite simply, it was his acceptance and knowledge of basic sciences as phenomena caused by forces within the natural world, where a plausible explanation regarding the source of disease could be found. Lister applied his scientific theories very well and solved the puzzle of surgical wound infections. Bugs or microorganisms were causing the surgical diseases, and it was absolutely required that they be eliminated when treating serious wounds.

Lister's Antiseptic Method

Lister's antiseptic method was not readily understood because it was very complex, according to many contemporary surgeons who were not used to painstakingly slow and delicate surgery. Surgeons were impatient and had, in general, no interest or knowledge of scientific principles. In reality, the routine application of science to surgery did not begin until the latter part of the 19th century, when pioneers like Halsted, the Mayos, Crile, Murphy, and others offered better means of cure and improved management.[14]

The complexity of Lister's method began with the use of antiseptics —
such as carbolic acid — that potentially eliminated the germs present in the
infected wound by washing, bathing, cleaning, and spraying the wound.
Instruments, surgeons' hands and the whole surgical environment were
also cleansed. For a great number of surgeons, this seemed unnecessary
since maintaining a clean wound was more than enough for them. There
was no incentive in the surgeons' professional career to advance the theoretical knowledge based on the germ theory of disease. Results were only
at the basis of their comprehension and acceptance, since science was not
considered in their approach to wound treatment.

Lister required that every element associated with the surgical act,
directly or indirectly, comes in contact with the antiseptic compound in
many forms, so that assurance could be given to all elements involved
regarding the absence of infection. Lister was absolutely convinced of the
virtues of antiseptics in preventing surgical wound sepsis. For Lister, the
antiseptic method was simple to understand, based as it was on the germ
theory of disease. Germs had to be eliminated at all cost. Since other surgeons did not believe in the germ theory, they were not pressured to
accept the use of antiseptics and, indirectly, the germ theory. Today it is
quite easy to correlate germs with disease, but this connection was much
less obvious to practicing surgeons who typically lacked scientific
involvement.

Lister's antiseptic method was scientific. All principles were explained
through well-designed objectives and demonstrated results, which were better than the results observed without antiseptic principles. Lister's method
rested on theory, a hypothesis, clear aims and, finally, well-carried out results.
There was no doubt as to the characterization of the principles. A full proof
of correlation existed among microorganisms, surgical disease and antiseptics.
The whole thing had been sealed from the scientific point of view. Lister had
reached the summit of surgical inquiry and had presented a new perspective
on the treatment of surgical wounds. A real surgical revolution!

Conclusion

Lister culminated his extraordinary work with the full acceptance of his antiseptic method. In spite of his well-recognized advances in the treatment of

contaminated wounds as we know it today, it took many years and even decades before everyone fully accepted his method.

Today we look back and realize the unique contribution of Lister to the progress of surgery, appreciating its full impact. Today we admire and cheer the clarity of his findings and the conception of a surgical revolution!

References

1. Lister J. (1867) On a new method of treating compound fractures. *Lancet* **1**:326.
2. Lister J. (1909) *Collected Papers*, 2 Vols. Clarendon Press, Oxford.
3. Toledo-Pereyra LH, Toledo MM. (1976) A critical study of Lister's work on antiseptic surgery. *Am J Surg* **131**:736–744.
4. Toledo-Pereyra LH, Toledo MM. (1979) Anticontagionism in the opposition to Lister. *Curr Surg* **36**:78–87.
5. Toledo-Pereyra LH. (1990) Joseph Lister: fundador de la cirugia cientifica. *Cirujano General* **12**:197.
6. Toledo-Pereyra LH. (1992) El cirujano y la ciencia. El cirujano científico. Conceptos en su desarrollo y formacion. *Cirujano General* **14**:25.
7. Toledo-Pereyra LH. (1996) *Maestros de la Cirugia Moderna.* Fondo de Cultura Economica, Mexico.
8. Toledo-Pereyra LH. (2010) Birth of scientific surgery. John Hunter versus Joseph Lister as the father or founder of scientific surgery. *J Invest Surg* **23**:6–11.
9. Youngson AJ. (1979) *The Scientific Revolution in Victorian Medicine.* Holmes and Meier Publishers, Inc., New York.
10. Bettany GT. (1885, reprinted 1972) *Eminent Doctors: Their Lives and Their Work, Vol. II.* Books for Libraries Press, Freeport, NY.
11. Hale-White W. (1935, reprinted 1970) *Great Doctors of the Nineteenth Century.* Books for Libraries Press, Freeport, NY.
12. Godlee RJ. (1918) *Lord Lister. Second Edition.* MacMillan and Co., London.
13. Cheyne WW. (1882) *Antiseptic Surgery. Its Principles, Practice, History and Results.* Smith, Elder, London.
14. Toledo-Pereyra LH. (2010) Surgical Research III. *J Invest Surg* **23**:129–133.

9

Birth of Scientific Surgery: John Hunter versus Joseph Lister as the Father or Founder of Scientific Surgery

by Luis H. Toledo-Pereyra, MD, PhD

Pre-Hunterian Surgical Science

In the two centuries before Hunter, we encounter surgical personalities of the stature of Ambroise Pare (1510–1590), the notable French military surgeon, and Andreas Vesalius (1514–1564), the great Belgian anatomist. Both had considerable influence in the development of surgery. Both made well-recognized developments to the advancement of the discipline. Both brought a new way to understand surgery, the first one related to the care of surgical wounds and the use of antiseptics to improve wound prognosis in the time before the general acceptance and understanding of antiseptic practices, and the second, who introduced a rejuvenated approach to anatomy, with a greatly advanced characterization of all or most of the structures of the human body.[1–14]

Closer to Hunter's time, we find William Cowper (1666–1709) the distinguished British anatomist; William Cheselden (1688–1752), the admired English surgical master; Alexander Monro Primus (1697–1767), the respected Scottish surgeon and founder of the Edinburgh school; and

Percival Pott (1714–1788), the recognized London surgical practitioner, among other notable surgical personalities. These were some of the individuals who were influential and had a decisive force in the surgical arena of the English Pre-Hunterian days.

What did the surgeons before Hunter know how to do? How far would they go with their treatments? How would they be able to handle those patients with serious surgical complications? What was going on at the time that was so special? Were those times better than previous eras? How do we imagine that they functioned without anesthesia?

Surgery before Hunter was not better than immediately after him in the sense that significant limitations existed before and after his time. Surgeons before Hunter had some knowledge of anatomy because of its emphasis, though they did not know exactly what to do with that knowledge yet. They were able to care for wounds in only a limited way because the field of surgical infection management had not developed yet. Amputations and excision of tumors were more frequently performed, as well as extraction of bladder stones. Hernia repair was imperfect and surgery for peripheral vascular aneurysms had not reached levels of success in pre-Hunterian times.

Patients with serious surgical complications could not be handled in a manner that was acceptable and successful either before or immediately after Hunter. Surgery could occasionally help if it were appropriate to begin with. Otherwise, the results were irremediable and patients would succumb to surgical complications. It was not easy to avoid these complications. There were minimal surgical advances during Hunter's time when compared to previous eras. One could say that the status of surgery remained about the same. Let us now review in more detail Hunter's contributions to surgery.

Surgery During Hunter's Epoch

John Hunter lived in the 18th century and therefore his contributions to surgery should have been more apparent by the end of the century or the beginning of the following one. No new procedures or techniques were introduced by Hunter, except for high femoral ligation for the treatment of popliteal aneurysms.[2] Otherwise, I could not find any other development, innovative enough, within the realm of surgery and its clinical application.

Perhaps his work on gunshot wounds, although not original, is worth mention. This work was not scientific in nature. Hunter did not sit down and carefully and systematically plan well-conceived surgical questions that would provide appropriate scientific answers. He did not study surgical disease and then execute a scientific plan that would provide him or others with definitive answers. He was extremely inquisitive and impulsive in searching for problems, but mostly outside of the surgeon's environment, and those related to surgery lacked scientific development.

As his professional life moved ahead, Hunter was a "reluctant surgeon"[2] and did not want to operate unless it was absolutely necessary. "Aversion for operations" was a phrase sometimes used when referring to Hunter's interest in the operating room.[2] Pertaining to his contributions to biology, anatomy, physiology and pathology, however, the results were completely different. Hunter extensively studied the human teeth, child development, the nature of digestion, venereal diseases, inflammation and the importance of lymphatics.[3] These particular studies, however, did not include surgery and they were performed because of his personal inclination to these individual matters without particular consideration for the scientific improvement of surgical practice.

Did Hunter utilize the surgical sciences in his surgical practice or in the evolution of his ideas? It is clear to me that Hunter did not apply science to the surgical field, but rather he remained on the outskirts of scientific surgery without implementing some of the observational findings from his own animal experiments. In point of fact, Hunter was not doing animal experiments to advance surgery. He was doing them because of his inborn and extensive curiosity in biology and its related fields. Hunter was advancing his own interests and quenching his stubborn thirst for knowledge, but surgery was in the background and did not represent his main field of scientific inquiry.

The intense interest of Hunter in anatomy stands in contrast to his feeble commitment to surgery. He moved from the reluctant surgeon to the assertive anatomist. He began dealing with anatomical works at an early age, probably because of his brother William, who was already working in this field in London.[1-6] In 1748, John Hunter joined his brother in teaching anatomy. He performed many of the preparations needed for the class, and handled all the details of student registration as well as requirements to carry out a good class, which initially had been cared for by William.[2] Under these arrangements the brothers remained together for 11 years. The anatomical school had moved from Covent Garden (1746–1760) to Litchfield Street (1763–1767) and finally to Windmill Street (1768–1783).[1,2] In our own account, we see John leaving William by 1759 because of health-related issues. With the intention of recovering in airy, open spaces, he enlisted in the British military and participated in the Seven Years' War with France.

In spite of William's desire to keep John at the school, a personal disagreement about the primacy of the discovery of blood supply to the placenta separated them for the rest of their lives.[1] Three years after this event, in 1783, William died and John expressed his inconsolable regret for not re-establishing contact with his brother.

"But Why Think? Why Not Try The Experiment?"

It is said, that when Edward Jenner (1749–1823), Father of Vaccination and a pupil of John Hunter, asked his master how to deal with certain medical or biological problems, Hunter immediately exclaimed, "But why think? Why not try the experiment?"[2–5] Hunter's attitude, even though experimental, was not scientific in the sense that he did not systematically study the question being asked. However, he did show significant inquisitiveness, interest, and desire to learn but not necessarily adopting the strict path of scientific inquiry. His approach was one of an experimenter who tries one or two times but does not repeat the same phenomenon as many times as necessary to reach scientific truth.

When we examine surgery, Hunter did not introduce a new scientific development in the discipline. While it was true that the high femoral ligation of popliteal aneurysms was a new and interesting concept, it was also devoid of science. Indeed, Hunter did not conduct surgical scientific research at any time during his career. His work was in areas separate from surgery and associated with medicine, such as infectious diseases in the case of syphilis and gonorrhea, and biology in relationship to inflammation, coagulation, and many other important concepts.

Hunter represented someone interested in many disciplines at the same time, particularly in questions that he could tackle aggressively and obtain

prompt answers for. Science as we see it today was not present in his surgical treatments, but could be better characterized through his biological
studies. He was curious and his trips allowed him to study areas that were
dear to his heart, such as animal anatomy and physiology, inflammation
and coagulation.

What About Lister, His Life and Surgical Ideas?

Joseph Lister (1827–1912) was a man ahead of his times. He took surgery
under his wings and moved the field to heights never reached before. As
opposed to Hunter, Lister had a great deal of support from his well-to-do
family. His father was Joseph Jackson Lister (1786–1869), who in addition
to being a wine merchant, was also the discoverer of the importance of
achromatic lenses in optic visualization, for which he earned entrance into
the Royal Society in 1832. There is no question that the Society gathered
the most celebrated scientists of its time. His son, Joseph Lister, was elected
to the Royal Society in 1860 at the age of 33 because of his "reputation as
an original and thorough investigator."[7] Almost one hundred years before,
in 1767, John Hunter had been accepted into the same illustrious group
because of his zoological studies on the greater siren at the age of 39 years.[7]

Joseph Lister had excellent early schooling and better formal education at the university level than John Hunter, who had none. Lister
attended medical school at University College, London, whereas Hunter
did not receive any formal medical school training except for isolated
surgical classes received at St. George, St. Bartholomew, and Chelsea
Hospitals. Lister had as mentors committed researchers, such as Wharton
Jones, renowned ophthalmic surgeon and a well-known student of
inflammation, and famous physiologist William Sharpey who advised
Lister frequently about his future career. Hunter did not encounter this
kind of support, inasmuch as his brother William was trying to cover these
missing elements.

Lister produced and published early, and by the end of medical school
he had already written many research papers associated with the use of the
microscope lenses invented by his father. Hunter did not have this extraordinary opportunity, except for working with his brother William in the
dissecting room.

At the suggestion of professor Sharpey, in 1853, Lister visited James Syme, the professor of surgery at the University of Edinburgh, for one month. Syme, by many accounts, was considered "the most original and thoughtful surgeon of his day."[7,11–13] This visit would change Lister's life. Firstly, professor Syme invited Lister to undertake what would be today's equivalent of a full surgical residency. Secondly, both of them, Syme and Lister, faithfully accepted and respected each other. Thirdly, in 1856, Lister married Syme's eldest daughter Agnes, which would be the highlight of his personal life and would cement his already good relationship with his teacher. Fourthly, his experience at Edinburgh would open doors for him. Hunter did not have the same experience, since his relationship with his mentors was not as close as Lister's to Syme, who eventually became his father-in-law. Hunter, however, like Lister, married well and into a medical family. Anne Home, his wife, was the daughter of Robert Home, an army surgeon, and his brother-in-law was Everard Home, a surgeon who later studied under Hunter and became close to him. Sadly, in 1823, Home burned Hunter's manuscripts in "a fit of jealous rage."[2]

In 1860, at the insistence of professor Syme, Lister accepted the Regius Professorship of Surgery at the University of Glasgow. By then, Lister had several significant scientific studies under way concerning the coagulation of blood, the early stages of inflammation, the structure and function of nerve fibres, the regulation of the contraction of arteries, the function of visceral nerves, the involuntary muscle fibers, the flow of lacteal fluid in the mesentery of the mouse, and other worthwhile scientific experiments. Lister was fully committed not only to clinical surgery but to research development as well. This full life, centered on surgery and research, never wavered.

Lister Develops His Antiseptic Theory

By 1860, Lister had begun to recognize the association of filth and unsanitary conditions in the hospital wards with excessive mortality. In the wards of the Glasgow Royal Infirmary, hospitalism was rampant, and translated into diseases like septicemia, erysipelas and pyemia. What to do next? Lister was overwhelmed by the unacceptable mortality — near 50% — that characterized all hospitals in Europe. These unacceptable figures demonstrated that something new and special needed to be done. But what? Lister tried to understand this very real problem without any good answer at the beginning.

The great awakening began in 1865 when Thomas Anderson, professor of chemistry at the University of Glasgow, alerted Lister to the great works of the genius French chemist Louis Pasteur.[7] In his brilliant experiments Pasteur wrote of putrefaction, fermentation, living microorganisms, dust and air as having a direct relationship with one another. In his own reports, Pasteur recognized that putrefaction was a fermentative process due to living microorganisms present in dust and transported by air. A year before, in 1864, Lister had become aware that carbolic acid had destroyed entozoan that infected grazing cattle at the sewage property of Carlisle. Immediately thereafter, Professor Lister developed his own antiseptic theory based on Pasteur's findings, as well as on his own experiments. Now, Lister had to prove that wound sepsis behaved and responded to treatment with some form of carbolic acid. The experiments would have to be carried out on patients.

In August 1865 the human experiment began! The results were evident and extraordinary since nine of 11 cases of compound fractures of limbs recovered. Even though Lister's system was complicated in its implementation, he had demonstrated that antisepsis was effective and that germs were the source of infection and its associated mortality. The germ theory of disease had been fully proven under these conditions. By 1867, when Lister's first paper was published in *Lancet*,[10] he had recognized the value of antisepsis, the value of Listerism. The science of Pasteur and Lister had triumphed in its application!

Further Studies by Lister into the Surgical Sciences

After publishing his classic paper of 1867 in *Lancet*,[10] one of many he would eventually publish, Lister moved ahead with more experiments and publications on this important area of unique surgical consideration. There is no doubt that Lister was adamant to prove his surgical antisepsis with actual cases, since he knew his findings were real and supported his innovative position. Many invitations and acceptances resulted and because of them he had the opportunity to travel throughout Europe and America.

His lectures were solid, well-organized and very didactic, reflecting his dedicated science behind his surgical remarks, highlighting his understanding of the germ theory as applied to surgery.

In 1869, Lister had the great opportunity of returning to the place where his father-in-law, James Syme had taught him the practical principles of surgery, where he had met his wife, and where he had so many followers and students, the great University of Edinburgh. This time he was returning as the chief of clinical surgery to occupy the position that Syme had held years before. This was in many ways a great personal triumph that culminated with returning to this praised city.

During his Edinburgh period, Lister researched and published about the ligature of arteries using the antiseptic system, the effects of the antiseptic system of treatment upon the salubrity of a surgical hospital, a method of antiseptic treatment applicable to wounded soldiers, the contribution to the natural history of bacteria and the germ theory to fermentative changes, the relation of microorganisms to disease, lactic fermentation and its bearings on pathology, and several other topics.[7,10]

In 1877, Lister received the last appointment of his career as chair of clinical surgery at King's College University Hospital, London. By this time, his research had diminished but not his deep commitment to disseminating the message about the application of antisepsis to surgery according to the germ theory. His published works during this period included familiar topics, such as the nature of fermentation, the relation of microorganisms to disease, the use of catgut ligature, the application of new antiseptic dressings, the principles of antiseptic surgery, the antiseptic management of wounds, the value of pathological research, the relations of clinical medicine to modern scientific development, and the value of antisepsis in clinical surgery.

By 1893, at the age of 66, at the end of his clinical and operating career, Lister had begun to close the doors of his private practice, laboratories and frequent social gatherings. During this time, his dear wife and close companion for 37 years, Lady Lister, contracted pneumonia while in Italy and passed away four days later. Her death created an incredible vacuum in the personal life of the great surgeon master. He accepted his destiny in public, although in private frequently mourned his wife.

From 1893 to his death in 1912, Lister was invited to the most prominent British medical and scientific positions of the time and he received a large number of honors in Great Britain and the rest of the world. A long life well lived!

Who is the Father of Scientific Surgery?

There is no question in my mind that Joseph Lister should be considered the "Father of Scientific Surgery." Some or many of you might disagree with me and consider John Hunter, the dignified surgeon, as worthy of this title. I think, through this writing, I have exposed the reasons behind my assertion and a comparative analysis of your own should help you in reaching the best conclusion.

Take into consideration that both men lived during different historical periods, Hunter in the 18th century and Lister in the 19th century. This mere fact should imply that Lister had more opportunities than Hunter for using more sophisticated thinking or support on the development of his science. Other than this, the rest has been explained throughout this writing.

Of primary importance is the fact that Lister applied all his work to practical cases, beginning with his first publication on the antiseptic system in 1867 and throughout his detailed examination of scientific method. He did not let go in terms of studying, reviewing the science again, analyzing everything he could in regards to this antisepsis system, proposing better ways to understand it, giving lectures on its virtues, demonstrating its beneficial effects and showing the positive results. Hunter, however, did not have a surgical scientific method or proposal to present or to move forward. All his scientific studies were outside the surgical arena. Since Hunter was an anatomist and inflammation biologist concentrating on infectious disease, he was not necessarily trying to apply anything to the surgical field. He did not introduce into surgery a well-thought-out scientific study. Many of the previous reasons are the basis for my current conclusion. I hope the reader can discern a personal view pertaining to the ownership of the title, "Father of Scientific Surgery."

Personal Remarks

I have always been an admirer of Joseph Lister since my early years at the University of Minnesota in 1972 when I encountered the lectures of

Dr. Leonard G. Wilson and the writings of Dr. Owen H. Wangensteen. Both of them were highly informative and stimulated my curiosity to begin my search for a better understanding of the contributions of the famed British surgeon to the surgery of his times and of today.

As I began my first studies on Lister, I encountered the help of Marjean, my wife, who gave her time and a sense of succinctness and practicality to the historical review of Lister's accomplishments. We both enthusiastically analyzed the impact that Lister had on the world of medicine and surgery. We ended up with impressive and interesting developments.[15]

As I completed my residency in surgery at Minnesota, in 1976, I presented my graduating lecture on the life and accomplishments of the great surgeon master, Joseph Lister. From then on, every time I could, I referred to his figure and personality to explain the advances of surgery based on his antiseptic method. Lister had a long lasting effect on my view of surgery and offered a new perspective to my discerning attitude.

From 1976, when I left Minnesota, to 1989 during my last year at Detroit's Mount Carmel Mercy Hospital, that is for 13 years, I did little to explore Lister's life and developments. However, I later took this message to Spanish speaking countries like Mexico, where I presented and published various papers on the outcome of Lister's works on the evolution of surgery. Even then, I brought for the first time the idea that Lister should be considered the "Father of Scientific Surgery."[14] Several papers and chapters emanated from these presentations and studies.[14]

I encountered another personal hiatus of more than 10 years in my dedicated attention to Lister until now, when I am focusing again on why Joseph Lister instead of John Hunter should be considered the "Father of Scientific Surgery." I hope that my concepts and ideas offer certain evidence of my logical and historical reasoning.

References

1. Dobson J. (1972) John Hunter. In: *Gillespie's Dictionary of Scientific Biography.* Vol. VI, Charles Scribner's Sons, New York, pp. 566–570.
2. Moore W. (2005) *The Knife Man: The Extraordinary Life and Times of John Hunter, Father of Modern Surgery.* Broadway Books, England.

3. MacCormac W. (1899) The Hunterian oration on Hunter as the founder of scientific surgery. *Br Med J* **1**:389–395.

4. Foster M. (2009) John Hunter: Founder of scientific surgery. *Endocrine Today* Vol. 7 **13**:1–9.

5. Ellis H. (2005) Book review. The knife man: The extraordinary life and times of John Hunter, father of modern surgery. *Br Med J* **330**:425.

6. Sheldon GF, Kagararise MJ. (1998) John Hunter and the American School of Surgery. *J Trauma* **44**:13–40.

7. Turner GL'E. (1973) Joseph Lister. In: *Gillispie's Dictionary of Scientific Biography*. Vol. VIII, Charles Scribner's Sons, New York, pp. 399–415.

8. Lister J. http://nndb.com/people/597/000091324/. Accessed November 17, 2009.

9. Lister J, 1st Baron Lister. http://www.newworldencyclopedia.org/entry/Joseph_Lister. Accessed November 17, 2009.

10. Lister J. (1909) *The Collected Papers of Joseph, Baron Lister.* (A facsimile of Collected Papers first published in 1909.) Classics of Medicine Library, Birmingham, AL.

11. Truax R. (1944) *Joseph Lister: Father of Modern Surgery.* The Bobbs-Merrill Company, Indianapolis.

12. Godlee RJ. (1917) *Lord Lister.* Macmillan, London.

13. Leeson JR. (1927) *Lister as I Knew Him.* London. Bailliere, Tindall, Cox, London.

14. Toledo-Pereyra LH. (1996) *Maestros de la Cirugia Moderna.* Ed. Fondo de Cultura Economica, Mexico.

15. Toledo-Pereyra LH, Toledo MM. (1976) A critical study of Lister's work on antiseptic surgery. *Am J Surg* **131**:736–744.

X-Rays Surgical Revolution

by Luis H. Toledo-Pereyra, MD, PhD

Introduction

In 1895, Wilhelm Conrad Roentgen (1845–1923) discovered X-rays, a new wonder for investigating the human body. No machine before had been able to demonstrate details of anatomy in the manner that Roentgen was bringing to bear.[1–15] The powerful aura of this particular discovery had no historical precedence in the world of medicine and surgery, but x-ray imaging equaled the introduction of anesthesia in impact. The assumption that the invention of the X-rays and related technologies created a surgical revolution is the tenet of this historical analysis.

Scientific Work Prior to Roentgen

Several scientists had been working on cathode rays prior to the work of Roentgen. Cathode rays constituted the principal source for the emission of X-rays, and the Crookes tube was the air vacuum container where the cathode rays were formed. These rays arose from a beam of electrons traveling from the negatively charged end to the positively charged end of the tube.[1,5] The emerging science of electricity had added a great deal to the understanding of the basic principles of physics demonstrated in the cathode rays and the creation of air vacuum tubes. In this regard, Franklin,

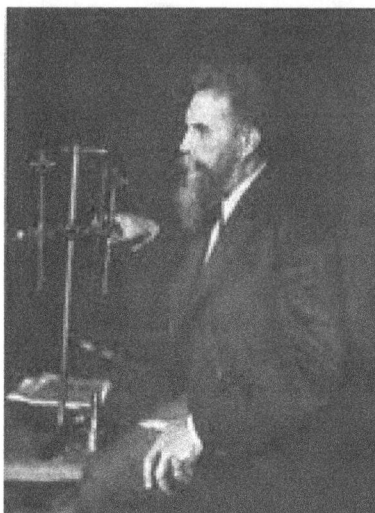

Figure 10.1.   Wilhelm Roentgen (1845-1923) at the Institute of Physics at the University of Munich in 1906.

Galvani, Volta, Faraday and Ampere made significant contributions.[1,2,5] Following their discoveries, Plucker, Hittorf, Varley, Goldstein, Crookes, Hertz and Lenard were the immediate benefactors of the advanced principles of electricity, and they directly applied the principles to the conceptual function and characterization of cathode rays.[1,2,5]

A basic understanding of electromagnetism existed as well. Its use, however, was not well defined and few scientists were applying it to the medicine of the time. All the knowledge accumulated up to this point did not represent a direct path to the discovery of X-rays. Roentgen's ingenuity and genius were necessary to combine all of these known factors in the world of physics, necessary to see clearly through previous work and apply it in a new, different and creative way. The capability of a scientific revolutionary was required!

Roentgen's Discovery

In 1895 Roentgen was concentrating on the study of the response of vacuum tubes when an electrical current passed through them. Years before at Strasbourg, he had been interested in several physical science problems,

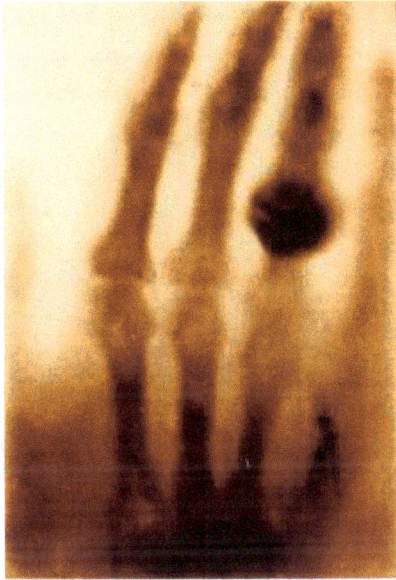

Figure 10.2. Hand radiograph of Roentgen's wife in 1895.

such as the ratio of the specific heat of gases, the conductivity of heat on crystals, and the polarization of light in gases. He took up the relationship between light and electricity while at Giessen, and later on, while at Wurzburg, he began to study the effects of pressure on the properties of solids and liquids and the importance of factors associated with cathode rays, vacuum tubes and electricity.[5]

On November 8, 1895, Roentgen was mulling over his observation of crystals of platinocyanide fluorescing when exposed to the effects of a Crookes tube.[1,2,5] What was happening? Was Roentgen expecting these findings? How could he explain this phenomenon?

Roentgen did not know exactly what was happening. He thought that a new force, a new ray was being produced. Roentgen did not expect these findings, as they were out of the ordinary and completely unplanned. There was no question that Roentgen was intrigued and decided to undertake further studies.

Roentgen repeated his initial experiments many times to ascertain the reality of the observations. Was this a fluke or was he seeing a very special

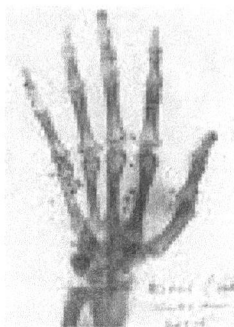

Figure 10.3.   Pieces of buckshot are seen in Prescott Butler's hand in 1896.

event, one never seen before? He asked himself these questions many times without a satisfactory answer. Roentgen believed in the virtues of constancy of purpose and commitment to his research studies and, thus, he persisted in continuously testing his findings.

This is the essence of his experiment: Roentgen took a black cardboard to cover a Crookes tube and attached electrodes to a Ruhmkorff coil (a generator) to produce an electrostatic charge. A fluorescent screen of platinocyanide received the images originating from the Crookes tube. The notoriety of this discovery exploded into the national and international news. All hospitals and universities desired access to the new technology. X-rays were not merely the patrimony of German medicine and surgery, but a boon to many other industries and countries. His discovery belonged to the world.

Wilhelm Roentgen's Life and Education

Wilhelm Roentgen was born in Lennep, Rhine Province, Germany in 1845, to a cloth manufacturer German father and a Dutch mother, and attended early school in Holland. He eventually moved to Switzerland to attend the Polytechnic at Zurich, where he graduated as a mechanical engineer with a PhD.[2]

Once he had moved to Germany, he started first as an assistant to professor August Kundt at the University of Wurzburg. Just about this time, he married Bertha Ludwig from Switzerland. Roentgen accompanied

Kundt to Strasbourg as a lecturer and later became a faculty member and professor. In 1879, Roentgen was appointed chair of physics at the University of Giessen, and in 1888 he was offered and subsequently accepted the chair of physics at the University of Wurzburg, where he was the director of the Physical Institute and in 1894 became the rector of the university.[2]

In 1900, Roentgen moved to the University of Munich at the request of the Bavarian government, assuming the chair of physics and became the director of the Physical Institute. By this time, Roentgen had enormous prestige and any university in the world would have wanted him as a faculty member. Roentgen was a recognized celebrity since his discovery of X-rays in 1895.

Six years later, in 1901, Roentgen received the coveted Nobel Prize in Physics, the first one to be given in this discipline to anyone "in recognition of the extraordinary services he had rendered by the discovery of the remarkable rays subsequently named after him."[11,12] The *world of science and later the medical establishment widely accepted this honor* and embraced Roentgen as one of the pioneers of medical discovery. Roentgen's unique perspective opened possibilities not previously considered, uncovering numerous potential applications.

Roentgen, a peaceful and kind man, remained reclusive as the years passed. He continued to pursue research, not on X-rays but in other physical science endeavors. His wife died of a long illness in 1919 and a year later he retired from his chair at Munich. His long country walks were legendary and he continued them until his death in 1923.

A Disconcerting Enemy of Roentgen and His Nobel Prize

Phillip Lenard (1862–1947), a well-known German physicist and discoverer of one of the cathode vacuum tubes, established a long-term feud with Roentgen and his 1901 Nobel Prize for the discovery of X-rays. Lenard felt that Roentgen had utilized one of his tubes but had not recognized his contributions to the discovery of X-rays.[1,5] Lenard vilified Roentgen and downgraded his role at every opportunity and to extraordinary lengths.

Lenard increased his criticism when he himself was awarded the Nobel Prize in 1905 for his work on cathode rays. He took the opportunity, at the Nobel ceremonies, to point out again that Roentgen had utilized his findings in obtaining the Nobel award, and claimed he had been overlooked at the time. Lenard's bitterness and resentfulness towards Roentgen were without precedent, and continued until his last interview in 1945, two years before his own death in 1947, and 22 years after Roentgen had passed.

Even though Lenard had introduced the cathode rays and been recognized for it, he believed "that the X-rays had been his baby and that Roentgen had been only the midwife, the mechanism of its birth."[1] The reality was that Lenard probably did not fully understand what Roentgen had done.

The successful combination of elements associated with Roentgen's discovery included many things besides the cathode tube discovered by Lenard, as well as similar tubes introduced by others like Crookes and many more. Roentgen discovered that, besides the cathode tube, other elements like the barium platinocyanide screen which gave a fluorescent glow, and the photographic plate, were required to produce the X-rays.

Did Roentgen Know the Impact that X-Rays Would Have on Medicine or Surgery?

Roentgen never realized the impact that X-rays would have on medicine or surgery. As a physicist, he did not know what was required for the application of X-rays in medicine or surgery. His interests were mainly related to research and its application in the physical sciences. When he took the X-ray of his wife, Anna Roentgen, as a demonstration of the effect of X-rays in uncovering the interiors of the human body, he did not know he had opened the new field of imaging with its profound implications for human anatomy, diagnosis and surgical approaches. He was inquisitive and eager to advance new developments but mainly as they pertained to physical phenomena, their fundamental operations, and explanations for those operations.

In this regard, Roentgen concentrated, in November and December of 1895, on moving forward the initial findings observed by Hertz and Lenard in the field of cathode rays research.[5] The power of cathode rays to produce fluorescence had been investigated by Lenard. Roentgen considered this to be a significant finding to which he would dedicate six weeks of his uninterrupted time.[1,2,5] That research established the difference between his studies and those of Lenard.

Roentgen approached the problem of cathode rays and fluorescence with different eyes and a different mind. He wanted to know what those rays were. How they propagated. How they refracted or reflected. What level of penetration they had. What tissues were they able to go through? How could one modify their movement? These and many more questions spurred his scientific curiosity.

Roentgen found that the new rays he had encountered were different from the cathode rays — they propagated horizontally and in a straight manner and were not showing refraction or reflection.[1,2,5] He also found that these new rays could traverse beneath surfaces and through dense material, imaging soft tissue and only stopping at bone. Roentgen knew at this point that he was facing a new ray that he labeled an X-ray.

First Clinical Uses of X-Rays

Roentgen first performed an X-ray on the hand of his wife Anna Bertha Ludwig Roentgen. Her hand bones were clearly photographed and amply visualized in a manner never seen before.[1] The resulting picture startled the world, permitting anyone to see inside the body. The public was awed. All around the world, scientists and laymen were attempting to use this incredible wonder. By the end of the 20th century, Friedman and Friedland named the discovery of the X-rays as one of the 10 most important changes in the world of medicine,[15] a well-regarded consideration not challenged by anyone.

After the unique demonstration by Roentgen, the second use of X-rays in humans and the first actual clinical case occurred a month later, when a German doctor requested their use on a young boy to diagnose sarcoma of the right tibia.[5] This was the beginning of the use of X-rays for clinical diagnosis. Doctors were eager to utilize this wondrous technique. Cases were piling up for diagnosis and follow-up of treatment. The question was how to obtain the machine that would allow physicians to demonstrate its benefit.

The third case followed soon after in the United States. This was the second clinical case in the world and the first one in this country. At

Dartmouth, New Hampshire, on February 3, 1896[4] Eddy McCarthy's left forearm Colles' fracture was imaged. Other cases followed and the positive results with the use of X-rays spread throughout the world like a fire. Everyone wanted to put their hands on the new discovery. X-rays had definitely arrived to make a durable statement in the diagnosis of medical and surgical disorders.

Other Technological Advances Based on the Discovery of X-Rays

Seventy-six years after the discovery of X-rays, CAT (computerized axial tomography) was invented in 1972 by British engineer Godfrey Hounsfield (1919–2004)[13] and South African physicist Allan McLeod Cormack (1924–1998), who at the time was at Tufts University.[14] Both of them, and rightly so, received the 1979 Nobel Prize in Physiology or Medicine.[12–14]

Other technological advances stimulated by the discovery of X-rays included ultrasound, which used sound and not light as the source of images. During the 1950's and beyond the number of scientists working on the effect of sound on imaging is too long to enumerate.[1] Suffice it to say that by the 1970's, the use of ultrasound in medicine and surgery was well on its way to becoming an established and well-respected diagnostic procedure.

Another gigantic step on the influence of X-ray technology on the investigation of the human body was the introduction of magnetic resonance imaging (MRI) in medicine and surgery. The 1980's saw this technology emerge with its diagnostic and awesome power in penetrating details of the human body that were previously not even imaginable. MRI studies were incisive and well-defined. MRI was something that X-rays alone could not equal in the diagnostic arsenal. MRI invaded anatomical regions that were out of reach of previous diagnostic techniques.

Nuclear medicine, PET (positron emission tomography) and SPECT (single photon emission computed tomography) are some of the new techniques that allow for functional organ visualization.[1] They were based on the use of radioisotopes, which originated in direct line from the initial acceptance of X-rays discovered by Roentgen. Analysis of the discovery of each one of these innovative medical advances cannot be addressed since they would require a more extensive study.

Other techniques, such as tomography and spiral CT are not discussed here either, because they represent variations of X-ray technology, which would deviate from our main concern of emphasizing X-rays and their role in a surgical revolution.

It was evident that by the 1990's, the field of X-ray application and technology had already advanced so much that the human body was being explored in unparalleled detail. X-rays by then had become a continuous positive ally of many surgical and medical specialties and permitted these particular fields of medicine and surgery to refine their practice immensely. Today X-rays remain in the permanent armamentarium of the medical and surgical specialties.

X-Rays Surgical Revolution

The influence of the discovery of X-rays on the development of surgery is without parallel when compared with other advances in the surgical profession. In fact, one could strongly assert that surgery would not be the same without the opportunities X-rays brought to bear. Roentgen never thought that the intriguing rays he had discovered were about to change the face of surgery specifically and the spectrum of medicine generally.

Having X-Rays available for more patients since 1896 allowed the surgical profession to utilize them first in the orthopedic surgical arena, where the diagnosis of broken bones and response to treatment with appropriate alignment were essential to managing patients. Other important anatomical sites, like the chest and the skull, were the next frontier for the practicing surgeon. Chest X-rays permitted the assessment of tumors, evolution of diseases like tuberculosis, discovery of fluid collections, and many more diagnoses. In the skull, the presence of fractures, opaque foreign bodies, the existence of hydrocephalus, and the characterization of pituitary tumors were the entities better identified with this technique.

As the knowledge of the potential of X-rays on surgical diagnoses became more apparent, other anatomical structures began to be explored, including the abdomen. Imaging of small bowel obstructions, the arrangement and characteristics of intra-luminal and extra-luminal gas, the spontaneous presence of air in the peritoneum, the identification of gallstones or renal calculi, the consideration of tumor masses with evident calcifications and the clear visualization of the psoas muscle bilaterally were all part of the basis for improving the diagnosis of the surgical abdomen.

Many other discoveries emanated from the simple application of X-rays. For example, the use of oil as a contrast material, the use of air in certain cavities to enhance the radiological exposure of neighboring organs, and the use of barium products to expose gastrointestinal structures made X-ray utilization more valuable. Other advances culminating in the use of ultrasound, CAT scan and MRI originated, at least in part, from the incredible wave of discoveries started by Wilhelm Roentgen, in the city of Wurzburg, on a Friday morning in November 1895.

In conclusion, it should not be doubted that the discovery of X-rays by Roentgen represented a real surgical revolution. Surgeons worldwide would not have been able to improve their art and science without the compelling photographic evidence of the organs they were operating upon. Professor Roentgen gave surgeons a diagnostic tool never dreamed of before and rarely equaled since.

References

1. Kevles BH. (1997) *Naked to the Bone. Medical Imaging in the Twentieth Century.* Rutgers University Press, New Brunswick, NJ.
2. Turner GLE, Roentgen WC. (1975) In: Gillespie CC (ed.), *Dictionary of Scientific Biography.* Vol. XI. Charles Scribner's Sons, NY, pp. 529–531.
3. Lentle B, Aldrich J. (1997) Radiological sciences, past and present. *The Lancet* **350**:280–285.
4. DiSantis DJ. (1986) Early American radiology: the pioneer years. *Am J Radiol* **147**:850–853.
5. Assmus A. *Early History of X Rays.* Obtained from: www.slac.stanford.edu. Accessed on August 1, 2009.
6. Donizetti P. (1967) *Shadow and Substance: The Story of Medical Radiography.* Pergamon Press, Oxford, England.
7. Gagliardi RA, McClennan BL. (1996) A history of the radiological sciences. *Diagnosis. Radiological Centennial.* Reston, VA.

8. Knuttson F. (1969) Roentgen and the Nobel Prize. *Acta Radiol Diagn* **8**:449–460.

9. Schwiertz G, Kirchgeorg M. (1995) The continuous evolution of medical x-ray imaging. *Electromedica* **63**:2–8.

10. Brecher R, Brecher E. (1969) *The Rays. A History of Radiology in the United States and Canada.* Williams and Wilkins, Baltimore.

11. Roentgen WC. Obtained from Nobelprize.org. Accessed on June 22, 2009.

12. X-rays. Obtained from Nobelprize.org. Accessed on June 23, 2009.

13. http://wikipedia.org/wiki/Godfrey_Hounsfield. Accessed on August 1, 2009.

14. http://en.wikipedia.org/wiki/Allan.McLeod_Cormack. Accessed on August 1, 2009.

15. Friedman M, Friedland GW. (1998) *Medicine's 10 Greatest Discoveries.* Yale University Press, New Haven, CT.

11

Concluding Remarks on the Surgical Revolutions

by Luis H. Toledo-Pereyra, MD, PhD

Surgical revolutions is the subject of this book in which we hope our intentions have been accomplished. That is to encourage those interested in history and the surgical sciences to review the origins of the discipline constructed from the perspective of a series of revolutions occurring in the history of surgery, in this case from the Renaissance period to the late 19th century.

If the clinician or historian can agree on the importance of the principles presented in this book, we can claim that this book has reached its highest potential.

The topics reviewed are self-explanatory, from Vesalius to Roentgen at the end of the 1800's. The advances throughout this period of history are well-established and need no explanation.

We encourage the reader to travel to the history of surgery with the same frame of mind we used when evaluating these events or individuals who transformed surgery into the discipline we know and enjoy today. We appreciate the reader's time and patience when evaluating our work.

SECTION II

HISTORY OF SURGERY AND MEDICAL HUMANITIES

Surgical Research II

by Luis H. Toledo-Pereyra, MD, PhD

Introduction

In our previous work on "*The Importance of Medical and Surgical Research,*"[1] we summarized our perspective of how research opened the doors for medical and surgical discoveries. Indeed, we said then that "without research the many advances encountered in medicine and surgery would not have been possible in the way we see them today."[1] In this writing, we focus exclusively on surgical research to continue our quest for better defining the origins of how research started to incorporate its principles into the surgical sciences.

We have selected a group of individuals who represent the beginning and early significant highlights of surgical research in the young American nation. In chronological order, we refer to William Beaumont (1785–1853), Samuel D. Gross (1805–1884) and William S. Halsted (1852–1922). Other great American surgeon pioneers who followed in their footsteps are not included in this writing.

Beginning Surgical Research in America

Since Galen's times in the first and second centuries, surgeons paid more attention to surgical skills and anatomy than anything else in the development of the discipline. As time passed, no significant changes were added to what was initially considered to be the critical aspects of knowledge and expertise.

During the Renaissance, Andreas Vesalius (1514–1567) introduced the final word in anatomical findings and can be considered the "Father of Modern Anatomy" for his enormous developments.[2] Even though Vesalius' contributions were unique for operating surgeons, research was not given attention in those times.

As for the American continent, in the American English colonies in the early 1600's research in surgery had no place whatsoever. The medicine of American colonial times was rather imperfect, with minimal understanding of surgery as we know it today. At the founding of the first American medical school, started in Philadelphia in 1765, surgeon-founder Philip Syng Physick (1768–1837) was a leading specialist in what would become the United States of America. However, he was not involved in research at any point during his illustrious career. Other medical schools were founded thereafter, but none brought surgical research to the forefront.[3]

William Beaumont, First Surgeon-Scientist

In 1785 when William Beaumont was born in Connecticut, surgery was still limited in its ability to cure and in its understanding of physiopathological processes. In 1822, when Beaumont, an established military surgeon, encountered the injured French-Canadian voyageur Alexis St. Martin, who had a gunshot wound to the left upper abdomen, he saw no hope for him. Beaumont thought St. Martin was going to die. To his surprise, St. Martin fully recovered. Only a small hole, the size of the tip of an index finger, was left after the wound healed. This gastric fistula gave Beamount full access to the human stomach and created a great opportunity for him (and later for all of us) to study the human gastric secretions in-situ.

How did Beaumont establish the best means to utilize this incredible opportunity efficiently and to realize one of the most important experiments in history? The exact details are not well-documented, but apparently Beaumont did not initially see the importance of this incident in terms of studying the gastric physiology in a human being.

We previously indicated in another publication that:

> "By early 1823, when St. Martin had fully recovered, Beaumont began to appreciate the special opportunity before him; the opportunity to study for the first time in the world the gastric physiology in a human being under direct vision; the opportunity to recognize changes that had never been reported in the medical world literature; the opportunity to make medical history."[4]

Beaumont began an exhaustive and systematic study of St. Martin's stomach secretions. Once Beaumont made his decision, he pursued St. Martin practically all his life. Beaumont performed 238 experiments in St. Martin's stomach and studied everything he could from the characteristics of the gastric juice in color, smell, temperature, changes of the food after passing the gastric secretions, and anything else he could encounter while doing the experiments. Beaumont also defined, with the aid of Dr. Dunglison from the University of Virginia, the existence of hydrochloric acid as part of the gastric juice.[4]

The ingenuity of Beaumont was evident, his ability to understand the process once it was perceived was unmatched, his persistence to reach some answers was beyond doubt, and his luck (under the circumstances mentioned with the full support of Surgeon General Joseph Lovell) was unique.

In 1833, Beaumont published his history-making book on the experiments and observations on the gastric juice, and created a special place for himself in the history of surgical research and the whole field of medicine in general. Because of his pioneering studies, Beaumont should be recognized as the "First Surgeon-Scientist of America" and most likely the rest of the world, and the "Father of Gastric Physiology."[4]

Samuel D. Gross, First Animal Surgical Researcher

After William Beaumont, no other American surgeon showed particular interest in clinical or basic research until Samuel D. Gross demonstrated his keen desire to understand how gunshot wounds exerted their injury, in other words to understand the mechanism of injury. Gross studied a series of animals — rabbits, cats and dogs — to define the characteristics and evolution of small bowel wounds. This was the first time that any American surgeon, or for that matter any American, was performing animal surgical experimentation.[5,6] Gross should be considered the "Father of Animal Surgical Experimentation" or "Father of American Basic Science Surgical Research."

A few years ago, I wrote about Gross:[6]

> "Samuel Gross was committed to surgical research in theory and practice. He devised and completed several basic research protocols when he was in Easton, later on at Cincinnati, and finally continued at Louisville…He posed theoretical and practical questions to the research performed in the three places mentioned above. Because of the pioneering surgical investigations initially carried out by Doctor Gross, before anyone else in this country, an appropriate title for him would be 'Father of American Surgical Research'."

After carefully reviewing the life and contributions of Beaumont and Gross, it is not simple to support my previous position and consider Gross the "Father of American Surgical Research" when Beaumont did systematic studies in a gastric gunshot wound in an adult individual for many years and published a book on the matter. Beaumont's studies were in humans and not in animals like Gross, but Beaumont did surgical research as well, even though of a clinical nature. So, to correct the previous title, I would like to re-emphasize, as indicated before, that Gross should be considered as the "Father of American Basic Science Surgical Research" instead, because he was the first animal surgical researcher in this country and before Gross, Beaumont was the first surgical researcher, although in humans alone. If we are to accept my explanation, Beaumont should ascend to the position of the "Father of American Surgical Research" in addition to the other specific considerations presented earlier.

William Halsted, Modern Surgical Researcher

In 1884 when Samuel Gross died in Philadelphia, William Halsted was still in New York and had not yet moved to Baltimore at the invitation of

William Welch (1850–1934), the noted pathologist in charge of organizing the academic faculty of the new Johns Hopkins Medical School.[7] Halsted had recently returned from a long European tour where he had visited and learned from some of the great old world stars. Billroth, Mickulicz, von Kolliker, von Bergmann and von Volkmann were some of Halsted's surgical masters, whom he visited for various periods of study in Europe.

Halsted learned everything he could from these great European surgeons. After having absorbed all the important successful characteristics of these masters, Halsted returned to the United States in 1880. He found a home at the Presbyterian and Roosevelt Hospitals, where he began his clinical research endeavors and became a well-known practitioner.[7,8]

In 1886, Halsted left New York to join Welch as they waited for the opening of the Johns Hopkins Medical School a few years later. Halsted's animal surgical research began at this time in the pathology laboratories of Dr. Welch. Halsted started by investigating the best principles for perfecting intestinal anastomosis techniques.[7,8] The project was long and required dedication, aided by Franklin P. Mall a future anatomy professor, who had come to join Welch in his laboratories and at the medical school. This interesting and worthwhile study would offer a great deal of help to Halsted, as the techniques moved to full clinical application.

More basic and clinical surgical research came along with the participation of Halsted's surgical residents, who had their own ideas to be tested in the surgical research laboratories. Basic and clinical surgical research was promoted by Halsted through the Hunterian Laboratory of Experimental Medicine, completed in 1905, on the surgical floors and in the operating theater.[8] Many pressing surgical questions were studied by Halsted and his disciples. From Harvey Cushing to Joseph Bloodgood, Jim Mitchell, John Finney, Samuel Crowe, George Heuer, Hugh Young, Walter Dandy and many others, the continuous input for solving important surgical problems was secured in Halstead's department of surgery.

A great number of research ideas were formulated and investigated in general surgery, endocrinology, urology, orthopedics, neurosurgery and many other surgical specialties, by notable surgeons who trained under Halsted. A new surgery was being molded and created under Halsted's leadership at Hopkins.

In conclusion, Beaumont, Gross and Halsted, at different points in the history of American medicine, represent the pillars of surgical research, and they are the pioneers to whom surgical investigation owes a great debt of gratitude.

References

1. Toledo-Pereyra LH. (2009) Importance of medical and surgical research. *J Invest Surg* **22**:325–326.
2. Sherzoi H. (2005) Andreas Vesalius (1514–1567). In: LH Toledo-Pereyra (ed.). *Vignettes on Surgery, History and Humanities.* Landes Bioscience, Georgetown, Texas, p. 44.
3. Toledo-Pereyra LH. (2006) *A History of American Medicine from the Colonial Period to the Early Twentieth Century.* Mellen Press, Lewiston, New York.
4. Toledo-Pereyra LH. (2005) William Beaumont (1785–1853). In: LH Toledo-Pereyra (ed.). *Vignettes on Surgery, History and Humanities.* Landes Bioscience, Georgetown, Texas, p. 58.
5. Toledo-Pereyra LH. (2007) Samuel D. Gross. In: LH Toledo-Pereyra (ed.). *Reminiscences on Surgery, History and Humanities.* Landes Bioscience, Georgetown, Texas, p. 109.
6. Gross SD. (1843) *An Experimental and Critical Inquiry Into the Nature and Treatment of Wounds of the Intestine.* Prentice and Weissinger, Louisville.
7. Toledo-Pereyra LH. (2005) William Halsted (1852–1922). In: LH Toledo-Pereyra LH (ed.). *Vignettes on Surgery, History and Humanities.* Landes Bioscience, Georgetown, Texas, p. 80.
8. Imber G. (2010) *Genius on the Edge. The Bizarre Double Life of Dr. William Stewart Halsted.* Kaplan Publishers, New York.

13

Arpad Gerster and Max Thorek Contributions to American Surgery

by Robert M. Langer, MD, PhD

"The twentieth century was made in Budapest," a 2001 article declared, describing the city as the birthplace of an improbable number of creative geniuses at the turn of the 20th century who made pivotal contributions in physics, chemistry, physiology, and literature.[1] The same Hungarian school system educated two other inventive minds — Arpad Gerster and Max Thorek — who immigrated to the United States and left lasting impressions on American surgery.

Arpad G. C. Gerster was born in Kassa, Hungary (today Kosice, Slovakia), on December 22, 1848, into a family of eight brothers and sisters. In this three-language city (Hungarian, German, and Slovak), the children received an impressive education, also learning Latin and Greek in school. Gerster later became fluent in English, French and Italian. As a boy, he enjoyed many competitive sports in addition to fishing, hunting, and tracking. He shared the family talent and passion for music, playing the piano and the organ. Two of his sisters sang professionally: Etelka became a celebrated soprano in the Milan Opera Company that toured Europe and the United States. One brother became a famous architect, another became a Professor of Chemistry at the University of Zürich. Gerster's interest in sketching and painting also began at an early age. In his autobiography,[2] he

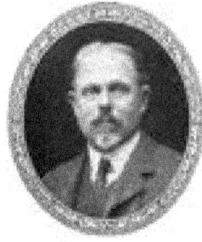

Figure 13.1.   Arpad G. Gerster (1848–1923).

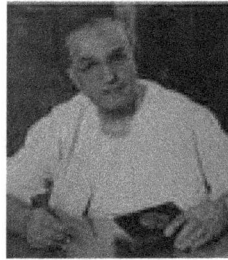

Figure 13.2.   Max Thorek (1880–1960).

fondly remembers his loving parents and his excellent, sometimes surprisingly liberal teachers from the Premonstrant order.

While Gerster dreamt of becoming an explorer or seaman, a friend who later became Professor of Urology at the University of Vienna, urged him to pursue a career in medicine. So Gerster chose to attend the University of Vienna Medical School. There he received perhaps the best medical education possible at that time. His teachers included anatomist Joseph Hyrtl, pathologist Carl Rokitansky, internist Franz Skoda, and surgeon Theodor Billroth, who later became Gerster's mentor. Billroth's charisma, intellect, and unflagging work ethic along with his rapport with his students, his calm manners and self-confidence in the operating room and his special cadaver courses taught to his assistants inspired young Gerster. Billroth's love for music, talent for playing piano, and friendship with Johannes Brahms represented other common interests.

During his years in Vienna, Gerster was an active member of the Hungarian Students Organization, which provided genial companionship, adventure, and an intellectual outlet. Following a duel, he nearly lost his fourth finger, which healed later with an interphalangeal ankylosis. He graduated in 1872 with a special diploma, i.e., Doctor of Surgery, which he earned by taking additional clinical courses and examinations. A year of military service followed in Vienna. Although he was offered a military post as a surgeon, Gerster already had other ideas for his future — to try his luck in the United States. Before leaving Europe, he was invited to see Billroth perform the world's first laryngeal resection. He also visited Richard Volkmann's clinic in Halle, Germany, where the Listerian principles were being applied with extraordinarily good results for wound treatment. Gerster later described his astonishment at primary closures of amputation wounds. He arrived in New York in 1874 with a letter of recommendation from Billroth.

During the passage, he met Miss Anne Wynne, who had just returned from studying music in Stuttgart. Later they married, lived happily, and had a son. Both their son and grandson became surgeons (personal communication, Dr. Joseph Gerster, 2002).

Although Gerster started general practice on his arrival, later he became an attending surgeon at German Hospital, being the first doctor in New York to exclusively practice surgery.[3] Later, he was honored by an appointment to the staff of The Mount Sinai Hospital despite his non-Jewish origins. During his 34 years of service, he modernized the hospital's functions and services, introducing the rotation system of attendances, residents, and students. He proved to be an excellent diagnostician, drawing on his profound medical and surgical knowledge. His rounds were replete with colorful stories: he was beloved of his students and assistants.[4] The Mayo brothers visited him when in New York to observe his surgeries and learn about his postoperative protocols.[5] Will Mayo remembered Gerster's sound and original surgical judgment and valued his reluctance to perform unnecessary surgery.[6]

In perhaps his most interesting scientific paper, Gerster made the original observation that dissemination of cancer may be caused by surgery.[7]

Among 40 cases of mastectomy, including 34 axillary lymph node removals, not a single death occurred, due to his aseptic methods — these results being in stark contrast to the 16.5% mortality rate reported in the literature of the day. His enthusiasm for asepsis-antisepsis techniques were in contrast to the widely held belief that suppuration was necessary for wound healing. His book *The Rules of Aseptic and Antiseptic Surgery*,[8] published in 1888, sold a record number of 11,990 copies in three editions. Interestingly, he illustrated the book using his own photographs, an altogether new method at the time, and he refused to write a new edition, saying, "...the ostensible purpose of the book...had been abundantly fulfilled."[2] In his other publications Gerster described a broad range of surgical techniques, such as brain tumor resections, trauma operations, laryngectomy, plastic surgical procedures, and nearly all types of abdominal interventions. His other creative idea was the replacement of a damaged portion of skull with a gold plate.[9] He also published numerous articles on the history of medicine.

His recreational activities mirrored his restless soul and inventive mind. He befriended Native Americans in the Adirondack National Park, where he satisfied his enthusiasm for hiking, fishing, hunting, horse riding, and boating. Today, his etchings and paintings are among the collections of the New York Public Library and the Adirondack Museum at Blue Mountain Lake, New York. He continued to play the piano and organ, organized a string quartet, and frequently attended classical concerts and the opera.

He never forgot his Hungarian roots and served the immigrant community throughout his life. For this service he was awarded the Austro-Hungarian Empire's Francis Joseph Order in 1894; however, characteristically he returned it 12 years later in protest of Austrian policies repressing Hungarian rights of free speech.[5]

He was one of the founders of the American Surgical Association and served as its president from 1911 to 1912. He was also president of the New York Surgical Society and professor of clinical surgery at The Columbia University, New York. In 1923, he succumbed to cardiac failure at the age of 75.

Max Thorek was born in 1880 in the same Tatra Mountain region as Gerster. His father was a physician and mother a midwife. In his autobiography,[10] he remembers his childhood years with nostalgia, especially his first love, Fanny Unger, known as Fim. Because her parents were among the richest in town and Max was shy, hope of a relationship seemed remote. But they shared a common love for music, and he soon started playing violin regularly during musical afternoons at the Unger household. Their common interests turned into real love, and despite the fact that Max went to Budapest for undergraduate studies, their relationship remained alive. In 1897, when his brother Philip was killed in political rioting, the Thorek family immigrated to the United States.

Upon arriving in Chicago, the family faced the daily hardships of immigrant life. Thorek's father could not work as a physician without a license, and his mother, being a midwife, delivered babies of fellow immigrants for little monetary compensation. His main goals were to become a surgeon and marry Fim. He worked hard to help his parents, and at every opportunity he taught, translated, and accepted odd jobs while learning English. Hope came again through the violin: a Gypsy-style orchestra was organized in Chicago, and he accepted the invitation to join, finally earning a steady paycheck. Then another unexpected opportunity changed his life. He learned about the University of Illinois Rush Medical School's scholarships for members of its orchestra. He rushed, violin in hand, to apply. But at the interview Thorek realized to his dismay that the orchestra was seeking only a snare drummer, an instrument he had hated since childhood. Nevertheless, he immediately accepted the challenge, asking for the full tuition fee. An appointment was made for an audition, giving Max only three months to learn to play the snare drum. He practiced day and night and received instruction from his friends in the Gypsy-style orchestra. After his neighbors complained of the constant noise, he continued practicing in a hot, humid cellar. His perseverance bore fruit and after a phenomenal performance at the audition, he was accepted.

During his medical school years, Thorek remained active in sports and lived a simple life; he rode a bicycle borrowed from a professor and his only clothes consisted of his orchestra uniform. In spite of the difficulties and language barrier, he received his diploma in 1904. After a year of obstetrical internship, he started his practice in one of Chicago's poor immigrant neighborhoods, where at the time more than 40 languages were spoken.

Soon Fim arrived and another dream came true. They married and after a year had a son, who was named Philip after his late uncle. He became a successful surgeon and clinical professor at the University of Illinois (1906–1998). Thorek wrote about Fim with great love and admiration; in fact she supported him in every manner — managing his finances and helping him immeasurably to realize his dreams throughout his life.

By working among the immigrants, Thorek knew intimately the social, economic, and health-related problems of the poor. Throughout his career he worked to find solutions to these problems. Hard work improved his own financial situation, but his dream to practice surgery still remained unfulfilled as he could perform surgery only in different hospitals or accept assistants' jobs with little chance for advancement. Good luck struck again, this time in the form of a like-minded colleague, Solomon Greenspahn, 15 years his senior. In 1911, they founded the American Hospital with the principle of making "a hospital with a human atmosphere where the patient is a person rather than a case." With their connections finance was arranged and the 25-bed hospital began accepting patients.

Thorek's charming personality, linguistic talent, connections within the immigrant community, and friends from musical, literary, and entertainment circles helped him to expand his clientele rapidly. He gained notoriety for being a surgeon of "stars and satellites," treating such legendary patients as Buffalo Bill, Arctic explorer Frederick Cook, world-renowned Gypsy fiddler, Jancsi Rigo, actors, and Italian opera singers. Nevertheless, the poorest patients from Chicago's West side received the same quality care. Soon it became necessary to expand the hospital, and plans for a larger facility in another location were drawn up. Construction began immediately, but stopped suddenly due to lack of funding. But as happened so often in Thorek's life, a solution was found, and in 1917 the new building got started.

Like most surgeons, Thorek also tried not to operate on his own family members. But unlike most surgeons, he broke this rule twice. When his son experienced severe trauma of his finger, he faced the decision to amputate it — the accepted practice for such an injury. He took a chance and successfully replanted it and the wound healed primarily. On the second occasion, he operated on himself! In 1913, during a surgery he was injured by a needle; the ensuing infection quickly manifested into an abscess on the dorsum of his right hand and his forearm. Despite his colleagues' advice to amputate the arm, Thorek, assisted by Fim, opened the abscess using local anesthesia, and recovered from sepsis.

The 1920s brought financial success, but like many others, Thorek nearly lost everything during the Great Depression. Miraculously, American Hospital remained open during these difficult days, and all the employees continued to be paid.

Thorek established his own experimental laboratory for endocrinology research in the attic of his hospital, which led to the so-called rejuvenation operations, i.e., testicular and ovarian transplantations. However, when he realized that his experiments served no practical purpose, he summarized his experiences in a book.[11]

Through his experiments and publications, he established a network of international relationships, travelling widely to visit great physicians and surgeons of the day. In 1935, despite the political turmoil preceding World War II and opposition from his colleagues, he founded the International College of Surgeons in Geneva, Switzerland. Today, the organization thrives with 14,000 members in 113 countries.

His inventive and creative nature worked wonders in hospital and operating room. For cholecystectomy, he suggested that the back wall of the gallbladder be kept in the liver, dramatically reducing the bleeding and bile leakage. He was also the first to write a book about plastic surgery in English,[12] and worked to achieve wider acceptance of the specialty.[13] His method of breast reduction with free transplantation of the nipple remains the standard technique.[14] One of the most notable contributions to medicine was his highly successful book *Surgical Errors and Safeguards* (1932),[15] which has been reprinted for nearly 30 years. It served to remind generations of surgeons that every case is a new challenge, independent of previous experience and other similar cases. His textbook of surgery was also a great success, leading to the publication of a special war edition.[16]

What today would be called hobbies or relaxation, Thorek called "magic carpets," meaning the other half of life, active recreation. At the top of his list stood classical music, but beginning in the 1920s, he also became an avid, talented photographer. Never one for half-measures, he founded the Camera Club of Chicago and The Photographic Society of America, and also wrote two books on the topic. His comprehensive knowledge of literature was impressive as he read and wrote German, French, and Italian in addition to English and Hungarian. Another passion was the history of medicine and surgery. His views against euthanasia, his humanistic approach to medical and social issues, as well as his optimism and sense of humor led to many honors from international societies and governments. He received the Knight of Legion of Honors from France and was awarded by the American National Academy of Sciences. He was also honored by The Distinguished Citizen's Medal. He held Bulgarian, Venezuelan, Italian, and Mexican titles as well. But, as he wrote in his autobiography, he valued most the gratitude and love of his parents and his friendship with people.[10]

Thorek died in Chicago in 1960 at the age of 80 from cardiac disease. His obituary in the *Journal of International College of Surgeons* read, "Hail and farewell to a titan."[17] But the spirit of "Dr. Max" lives on: in 1975, the American Hospital changed its name to The Thorek Hospital, and Chicago's International Museum of Surgical Sciences was founded in 1952 at his bequest.

Both the above-mentioned surgeons were fantastic, but no saints. Gerster was not brilliant but rather a slow surgeon in the operating room and his humor would not be always appreciated today. Thorek had a very difficult relationship with the American College of Surgeons and that's why he founded the international organization. But the parallels in the lives of these great surgeons are astounding — solid education, knowledge of languages, talent for music, literature, and arts, creative thinking combined with hard work, good humor, as well as a social conscience. Clearly, these traits led both men to make groundbreaking contributions to American and international surgery.

References

1. Smil V. (2001) Genius loci. *Nature* **409**:21.
2. Gerster AGC. (1917) *Recollections of a New York Surgeon*. P.B. Hoeber, New York.
3. Rutkow IM. (1987) American surgical biographies. *Surg Clin North Am* **67**(6):1153–1180.
4. Baehr G. (1955) Profile of a surgeon. *J Mt Sinai Hosp* **21**:337–340.
5. Mayo WJ. (1925) Master surgeon of America. Arpad Geyza Charles Gerster. *Surg Gynecol Obstet* **40**:582–584.
6. Nelson CW. (1992) Dr. Arpad Gerster and the Mayo brothers. *Mayo Clin Proc* **67**:620.
7. Gerster AGC. (1885) On the surgical dissemination of cancer. *NY Med J* **41**:233–236.
8. Gerster AGC. (1888) *The Rules of Aseptic and Antiseptic Surgery*. Appleton, New York.

9. Gerster AGC. (1895) Heteroplasty for defect of skull. *Trans Am Surg Assoc* **13**:485.

10. Thorek M. (1943) *A Surgeon's World*. J.B. Lippincott, Philadelphia, PA.

11. Thorek M. (1924) *The Human Testis and Its Diseases*. J.B. Lippincott, Philadelphia, PA.

12. Thorek M. (1942) *Plastic Surgery of the Breast and Abdominal Wall*. C.C. Thomas, Springfield, IL.

13. Romm S. (1984) Max Thorek. *Ill Med J* **166**:331, 353.

14. Ruberg RL, Shah RR. (1983) Max Thorek: a surgeon for all seasons. *Clin Plast Surg* **10**:611–618.

15. Thorek M. (1932) *Surgical Errors and Safeguards*. J.B. Lippincott, Philadelphia, PA.

16. Thorek M. (1938) *Modern Surgical Technique*. J.B. Lippincott, Philadelphia, PA.

17. Editorial. (1960) Once in a lifetime: hail and farewell to a titan. *J Int Coll Surg* **33**:129–130.

14

Michael E. DeBakey: Reformer of Cardiovascular Surgery

by Roberto Anaya-Prado, MD, PhD, Eduardo D. Aceves-Velázquez, MD, PhD, Sara P. Carrillo-Cuenca, MD, and Luis H. Toledo-Pereyra, MD, PhD

Introduction

From time to time, in every career, there comes along a genius who revolutionizes the profession, and even the world, forever. Dr. Michael Ellis DeBakey is one such person. In cardiac medicine advancements, he is the undisputed pioneer of this century, maybe even in history. The creation of the ventricular assist device (VAD) and his many other firsts have revolutionized heart surgery (specifically aortic surgery) forever. He was a man who was given his own floor at the Baylor College of Medicine in Waco, Texas. Yet, to understand the full impact of this man, one must understand where he came from, what he did, and how he did it.

Meager Beginnings

"I have been asked what inspired me to take the path I have pursued in life. The answer lies in my boyhood. My parents, with their keen intellects, natural curiosity and high standards, were superb models... ."[1] What better tribute could be paid to one's parents? From their perspective, the

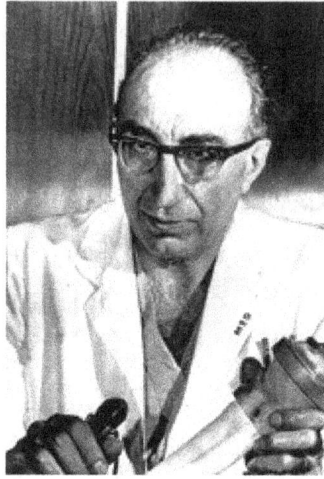

Figure 14.1.   Michael E. DeBakey (1908–2008) displaying an artificial heart at a 1966 press conference.

basic key to his success was proper parenting. It is quite obvious from this quote that DeBakey thought of his parents as one of his greatest resources for personal and spiritual growth.

DeBakey's parents were Shaker and Reheeja Zorba DeBakey. His mother and father were first-generation immigrants to the United States from Lebanon, settling down in Lake Charles, Louisiana, where DeBakey was born and raised.[2] His father pursued many different avenues for employment after he arrived in the United States. He once was a pharmacist running his own drugstore and, interestingly enough, this was DeBakey's first exposure to medicine. Shaker DeBakey also tried his hand at rice farming, real estate and construction. His parents, especially his mother, were deeply religious people, and raised DeBakey in the Episcopal Church. Thus, religion became a very important part of his childhood and of his spiritual growth as an adult. From this religious upbringing, DeBakey learned precious lessons such as a fondness for reading and studying, honesty, compassion, kindness and independence.[3]

Michael Ellis DeBakey was born on September 7, 1908.[4] As a child, DeBakey and his siblings, Ernest, Lois and Selma, were exceptionally bright.[2] As a young boy, he found the *Encyclopedia Britannica* to be fascinating and used to spend time at the library reading it. When he realized that he could not take it home, he told his father who, in turn, bought the entire set to have at home. When DeBakey and his siblings reached high school, they had already read the entire set. Later on, each one of them read one entire literature book per week, on top of their school work. William C. Roberts, who interviewed DeBakey in 1997, said that he calculated that Dr. DeBakey must have read 600 books between the ages of six and 17, to which DeBakey replied, "Yes, at least, plus the encyclopedia. I was a voracious reader."[4] All of the DeBakey children did very well in school, which led Michael DeBakey to skip a grade.[3]

When he was a boy, his mother taught the neighborhood girls to knit, cut a pattern and use a sewing machine. DeBakey found it so interesting that he learned the trades himself. He would later use this skill to sew the first Dacron artificial blood vessel. He was also quite a musically inclined child. His first instrument was the piano, and later on he learned how to play the saxophone. In college he joined the marching band and also learned how to play the clarinet, so that he could take part in the University's orchestra.[3]

> "We hear much today about the disintegration of the American family and my heart goes out to those who have missed the joys of belonging to a close-knit, loving family. I feel fortunate in having received moral and spiritual guidance as a child…Intellectual development without these values is compromised, in my view."[1]

Higher Education

After graduating from High School, DeBakey went to college at Tulane University; it was there that he earned his bachelor, medical and master's degrees. At first, he was not sure about becoming a surgeon, but encouragement from his mentor, Dr. Alton Ochsner, sent him down such a path. He completed his residency at Charity Hospital, in New Orleans. He then went to Strasbourg (France) and Heidelberg (Germany) Universities, by Dr. Ochsner's recommendation. In 1937, when he returned to the United States, he and Ochsner continued research and published the first article in which a link between smoking and lung cancer was noted.[5]

"In his senior year, DeBakey devised a modified roller pump that mimicked the heart's pulse wave. The roller pump would become the critical element of the heart-lung machine."[3] This invention began during his sophomore year in medical school where he worked as an assistant technician in a laboratory for another member of the faculty who was interested in the pulse wave.[4] Unable to find adequate information in the University's medical library, DeBakey immersed himself in the engineering library. He studied pumps dating back to two thousand years, using this information to manufacture his first heart pump prototype, which would become a reality only two years later.[2] "Modern heart surgery was born and DeBakey's career was just beginning."[2]

Tour of Duty

DeBakey was on his way to becoming a great surgeon. However, when World War II broke out, he found it necessary to volunteer for service. He was under no force or duress to do so, but chose to by his own will and volition. "DeBakey felt it was his duty to enlist at the outset of World War II, even though his colleagues at Tulane pleaded that he be declared 'essential' at the Medical School."[3] DeBakey replied, "When Fred Rankin, who was the Chief Surgical Consultant in the Surgeon General's Office of the Pentagon, learned... that I wanted to go into the service, he told Dr. Ochsner that he wanted me in his office."[4]

Working for the Surgeon General, DeBakey was able to spend much of his time reading and writing. His main job was to write down everything they did. While doing this he realized that the Surgeon General's National Library of Medicine, which was run and housed by the army, needed a new home and some help. The roof was leaking and there was too much information for that small room; everything was shoved together and packed too tightly (2). DeBakey realized that this priceless wealth of information needed to be preserved. He wanted to have a new library built in Washington, but was told that the army was more concerned about purchasing tanks than improving the library. "And that triggered in my mind suddenly, that it didn't belong in the army — it was a national treasure."[5]

He then proposed that it should be taken out of the army's hands and moved to a new location.[3] After the war, he was the driving force behind the bill in Congress that would allow the Library to be moved and taken out of the army's jurisdiction. Its purpose was to serve as a repository for medical journals and information so doctors could do research. Finally, the bill was passed through Congress in 1956. Senator Hill, who was one of the key men behind the campaign called Dr. DeBakey and remarked, "Mike, I don't know what you did, but we are going to get the Library bill through."[4] What DeBakey had done was to call in a favor. "Today the library has over 6.2 million books, journals, technical reports, microfilms and audiovisual materials."[3] The library is now the National Library of Medicine located in Bethesda, Maryland.[2]

Dr. DeBakey is also credited with developing the Mobile Army Surgical Hospital (M.A.S.H.). He wrote many papers and began to consider the idea that it would be much more advantageous for the soldiers if they could be treated closer to the battlefield, rather than being shipped to a far away hospital. "These M.A.S.H. units were an outgrowth of Dr. DeBakey's work at the Surgeon General's and these units saved thousands of lives in the war and in wars that followed."[3] Evolving from this project was a network of health services for the men returning from war. President Truman, in 1948, proposed for the Navy Hospital to be turned over to DeBakey to organize and take care of.[3] They offered immediate and long lasting care for all injured men returning from war. This is now known as the Veterans Administration and Veterans Affairs Medical Centers.[2] DeBakey also recommended for these hospitals to have an association with a medical school.[6]

Settling Down

After his military service, Dr. DeBakey returned to his medical career; it was 1948 and he was 40 years old. He was widely known for all the papers he had written for the Surgeon General and had his name widely publicized. He was considered one of the most promising new surgeons of his generation and had many job offers when he returned to the medical work force. After turning down three job offers in New York, he settled down as Chairman of the Department of Surgery in Houston at Baylor University College of Medicine.[4,6] DeBakey bought a house only five minutes away from the hospital. He wanted to save himself some time.

DeBakey logically comments, "I am a surgeon and if I get a call in the middle of the night, I don't want to use the telephone, I want to see the patient."[4] "After a disappointing start, DeBakey came close to declining. There were no residents or full time faculty and no teaching hospital."[6] Instead of resigning, he found a way to turn this around and, with the help of Mr. Ben Taub, he had The Jefferson Davis Hospital affiliated. He then enlisted the Houston Veterans Administration Hospital (now named Michael E. DeBakey VA Medical Center). Later in 1951, along with Ted Bowen, President of the Methodist Hospital, the latter and the Baylor University College of Medicine developed an important relationship through Dr. DeBakey.[7,8]

Throughout this decade, DeBakey did not neglect surgery. During the 1950's, DeBakey had many firsts: the first successful carotid endarterectomy (1953), the first successful resection and graft replacement of an aneurysm of the distal aortic arch and upper descending thoracic aorta (1954), the first successful resection with graft replacement of an aneurysm of the thoracoabdominal portion of the aorta between the chest and abdomen (1955), and the first successful patch-graft angioplasty (1958).[5]

In 1968 he was invited to be Dean of Baylor University and reform their way of doing things. Interestingly, DeBakey was later to save the University from financial ruin. In order to do this, DeBakey made the Baylor College of Medicine an independent entity from the Baylor University. With the help of a warm and supportive staff, he was able to raise more that thirty million dollars, which covered the college's financial deficit and saved it from bankruptcy.[4]

Dacron Artificial Arteries

A sewing machine does not seem like it could be a medical device, yet DeBakey was able to foresee its potential to be just that. His mother had taught him to sew as a child.[9] In 1953 he began working at home sewing an artificial artery made out of Dacron material.[3] So he went to a department store to buy some nylon, suggested as a possible alternative. The store was out of fabric, but the sales clerk suggested Dacron. DeBakey bought a yard of Dacron, took out his wife's sewing machine, and sewed a tube of the necessary size.[5]

The Dacron-velour material had never been used in this capacity before.[7] Later on that year, "He completed the first successful removal and graft replacement of an aneurysm."[3] An aneurysm is when the blood vessel's wall becomes weak and balloons out. The Dacron created an artificial blood vessel that could be grafted onto the existing blood vessel to prolong the patient's life.[8] Although it was a radical idea in 1953, "Such grafts are now part of a standard treatment."[9]

The LVAD

One of DeBakey's most acclaimed inventions is called LVAD or VAD, which stands for left ventricular assist device. "A ventricle assist device helps patients whose hearts aren't pumping sufficient blood to maintain adequate blood flow while either recovering from heart surgery, waiting for a heart transplant or for a host for other medical reasons."[10] It is made out of lightweight titanium and is about 1.2 inches long and 1.1 inches wide.[11] The initial idea and research for this device began in 1960. At that time, DeBakey said it was "highly controversial." Cardiac surgeons knew that the heart–lung machine was very helpful during recovery periods after a patient's surgery; however, they were quite skeptical about DeBakey's new VAD idea.[7] The first time this device was successfully implanted and used was in 1966. The VAD kept a 37-year-old woman alive long enough for her to be weaned off the heart-lung machine. From that point on, DeBakey's invention gained credibility. "This was the first successful case after 10 years of striving," Debakey said.[7] This was only the beginning for the LVAD.[10,12–14]

Space and Science Meet

DeBakey's work stretched far and wide in influence, even to NASA. In 1984 David Saucier, an engineer at NASA/Johnson Space Center, underwent a heart transplant. While Saucier recovered, it was proposed for NASA and DeBakey to team up to develop an implantable VAD. The first stage would be a temporary recovery device, then, eventually, a permanent implant. This application emerged from NASA turbo pump technology, in combination with NASA's computational fluid dynamics analysis capabilities.

To develop the high performance required for the Space Shuttle main engines, NASA pushed the state of the art in the technology of turbo pump design. Computational fluid dynamics software developed for use in the analysis of Shuttle external subsonic and supersonic flow was used in the miniaturization and optimization of a very small heart pump based on this new Shuttle technology.[10] An agreement was made between the Baylor University and NASA to work on the VAD project together.

At the time, there were two major concerns faced by doctors who were trying to create an artificial heart. The first was hemolysis, the second were thrombi. Using the NASA supercomputers, they were able to predict what would happen to the device as they changed one thing or another and saw how it would react: The DeBakey VAD pumps blood in a different manner than the natural heart. The VAD pumps blood with a rotating, screw like impeller (a device that forces liquid in a given direction under pressure) in a continuous flow, as opposed to the pulsed flow produced by the natural heart. "The VAD does not eliminate the pulse," DeBakey said. "The heart stays there... what's different is that the pulse is much stronger."[12] They ended up with a miniature device with only one moving part.

Debakey and Boris Yeltsin

In 1996 Boris Yeltsin was the president of Russia. He was having many difficulties with his heart. He was newly elected for his second period even though he had suffered three heart attacks in the previous two years. DeBakey was asked to take a look at him and give a prognosis. He convinced Yeltsin's doctors to postpone his heart bypass surgery for up to 10 weeks, arguing that Yeltsin needed recovery time before the surgery. However, DeBakey found out that his overall health was not as bad as many had thought.[14] DeBakey brought along his VAD device, just in case Yeltsin needed to become the first human patient to have one. Fortunately, or not, this did not happen.[2] Yeltsin is only one in a large list of DeBakey's famous patients. The Shah of Iran, the Duke of Windsor, Marlene Dietrich and Jerry Lewis are among others. Yeltsin is quoted as having said that "DeBakey was a man with an almost magical capacity to cure people."[2]

On a Personal Note

It had often been rumored that DeBakey had a temper and that he could be very difficult to work with. At Baylor University he was nicknamed the "Texas tornado." Dr. Noon, who had been a student and later worked with DeBakey for 30 years said, "DeBakey was good at getting everything organized, but delays and disruptions made him mad. Now his schedule is not as demanding and he is less high-strung."[9] When DeBakey was confronted with the question of his reputed temper he commented, "Maybe I should be more compassionate with people who do not think as fast as I can...I have little tolerance for incompetence, sloppy thinking and laziness." He had been quoted saying to young doctors, "You have four fingers and a thumb like I do. Why can't you use them the way I do?"[9] This came from a 90-year-old man who still practiced surgery.

Some would criticize DeBakey quite harshly, however. "No question, he has a pretty big ego," said Claude Lenfant, Head of the National Heart, Lung and Blood Institute, and then he added, "his contributions have been enormous, and he will leave an amazing legacy."[9] As one can see, even DeBakey's critics cannot deny the impact he has had on the world of medicine. In his early nineties, he still practiced surgery. At 90, a columnist wrote of him, "The ageless Dr. DeBakey, still cutting...He says he has no intention of retiring. He was recently pronounced as fit as most men far younger than him."[9] DeBakey was a man that accomplished all he set out to do. Michael E. DeBakey died on July 11, 2008. DeBakey improved the condition of life for so many people and the ideas behind his research continue even after his death.

References

1. DeBakey ME. (1987) In: PR Manning, L DeBakey (eds.). *Personal Essay. Medicine: Preserving the Passion*. Springer-Verlag, NY.
2. Sternberg S. (2000) The heart of a tiger: a cub named Karma tries to hang on till surgeons can save his life. *USA Today* Dec **07**.
3. Widmeyer R. (1998) A lifetime of imagination and dedication. *Texas Medical Center News* **20**:19.

4. Roberts WC. (1997) Michael Ellis DeBakey: a conversation with the editor. *Am J Cardiol* **80**(3):394–395.

5. Mitka M. (2005) Michael E. DeBakey, MD: father of modern cardiovascular surgery. *JAMA* **293**(8):913–918.

6. Noon GP. (2008) In memoriam Michael Ellis DeBakey, M.D. *ASAIO J*. **54**(6):559–562.

7. Larkin M. (1999) Michael DeBakey: taking challenges to heart. *The Lancet* **353**(9162):1420.

8. Christianson EH. (2000) DeBakey, Michael Ellis. *World Book Encyclopedia* **Jan 1**.

9. Altman LK. (1998) The ageless Dr. DeBakey: still cutting. *Detroit Free Press* **Sep 4**:5–6.

10. Dotts B. (2007) Ventricular assist device:(VAD or Heartpump). *NASA-JSC*. http://technology.jcsnasa.gov/techops/heartpum/heartpum.htm. Accessed in January 2007.

11. Bensch F. (1998) The DeBakey titanium heart assist pump. *Reuters News Pictures Service* **Nov 17**.

12. Dyson MJ. (1999) Have a heart. *Odyssey* **8**(6):27.

13. Nickolaus B. (1998) Hetzer, Noon and DeBakey implant new titanium heart assist pump in Berlin. *Reuters News Pictures Service* **Nov 17**.

14. MacFarquhar E. (1996) Prognosis improves for one Russian. *U.S. News & World Report* **Oct 7**:27.

15

Christiaan Barnard

by Luis H. Toledo-Pereyra, MD, PhD

Introduction

Christiaan Neethling Barnard (1922–2002) had a meaningful and complicated life. He contributed to the medical and surgical world by advancing the cardiac surgical sciences to the highest point possible with the realization for the first time of a successful human-to-human heart transplant. Barnard was a consummate academician and scholar who produced and reported some of the most notable cardiac surgical developments.[1–12] Barnard was a talented and gifted individual, who brought to his country, South Africa, and to himself the greatest accolades to be served upon a young country and a young surgeon, eager to be recognized and participate in the world scene. In this publication, I am interested in presenting the man, the surgeon, the scientist and the innovator.

Barnard the Man and His Education

Christiaan Barnard came from a low middle-class family from Beaufort West, in the Karoo region of South Africa. His father Adam and his mother Maria were dedicated religious people. The father, being the pastor of the Dutch Reformed church of Calvinist descent, initiated his family into his own religion. Maria played the organ at the church and cared

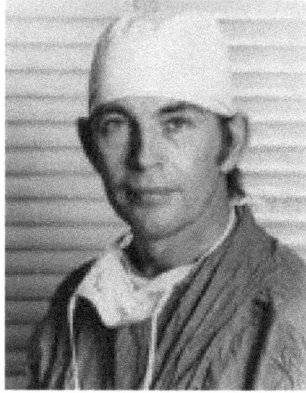

Figure 15.1.   Christiaan N. Barnard (1922–2002).

for all domestic activities. Five boys completed the family: Johannes (Barney), Dodsley, Abraham (who died at the age of four), Christiaan and Marius, in order of seniority. Dodsley was five years older than Christiaan and Marius was the youngest.[11]

Chris, as he was called by family and friends, grew up in a principled and God-driven, dedicated family where religion had originated from the Dutch colonizing the Cape of Good Hope area in 1652. They were Afrikaner Christians who accepted other races besides whites into their churches. Chris was never exposed to bigotry or anything like it during his early years of life. He learned to be tolerant, accepting, fair and under-standing. In later years Chris Barnard was described as hard working, intensely driven, motivated, perseverant, focused and self-confident.

After finishing at Beaufort West High School, Chris continued his studies at the University of Cape Town. In 1946, he graduated with the degrees of Bachelor of Medicine and Surgery (MB,ChB) from the University of Cape Town. Internships at Groote Schuur Hospital in Cape Town were secured from 1946–1948. During the last year, in 1948, he married Aletta (Louwtjie) Louw, a good looking nurse, whom he had met while in medical school. Two handsome children (Dierdre and Andre) and long separations were to come in a short few years ahead.

During the same year, in 1948, he moved to Ceres, Cape Province, where he practiced family medicine for several years. Perhaps these were the best years of his marital life, since he kept close to his wife and was at home more frequently. In 1951, he returned to Cape Town where he served as an internal medicine resident at Groote Schuur Hospital under professor Brock until 1953, when he took the Master of Medicine degree at the same university. That year he presented his MD thesis on "The Treatment of Tuberculous Meningitis" and entered the Department of Surgery as a resident at the same hospital for more than two years under Professor Erasmus. These were busy years for Chris, but happy in regard to worthwhile work. He enjoyed this period of his life as well and represented a dedicated and concentrated effort in obtaining a broad education in surgery.

In 1956, one of his dreams came true when he received the Charles Adams Memorial and Dazian Foundation Bursary for two years of study in the United States. This was a real opportunity for the young and aspiring Dr. Barnard. It is possible that no one else could have appreciated this scholarship as much as he did. The stage was set for him to begin his stint at the University of Minneapolis in Minnesota under the general tutelage of Professor Owen Wangensteen (1898–1981) and the direct mentoring of professors C. Walton Lillehei (1918–1999) and Richard L. Varco (1912–2004). These Cardiothoracic Surgeons received him with a positive and friendly attitude. For two-and-a-half years Barnard demonstrated himself to be one of the most dedicated and hard-working residents in the laboratory and surgical service. There was no rest for him, continuous hard work was his motto, and his mentor, the heart pioneer C. Walton Lillehei, referred to Barnard as someone with "intense ambition and ability to work" among many other virtues.[3,5,11] Lillehei, who knew his student for two-and-a-half years, longer than many other people, certified as to the character of the forming cardiac surgeon: intensively driven, extremely dedicated, very innovative, a man with a prodigious memory, but at the same time someone who was outspoken, self-confident, abrasive, arrogant and selfish.[11]

While at Minnesota, Barnard developed a close friendship with John Perry, another trainee under Wangensteen and Lillehei, and later Chief of Surgery at Saint Paul Ramsey Medical Center in St. Paul, Minnesota. Both surgeons-in-training then, Perry and Barnard established a better relationship than Barnard had with most people in America. Perry considered

Barnard a dedicated man, who was "driven to accomplish," innovative, skeptical, "impatient and hoping to reach something noteworthy."[11] Both enjoyed each other's company and remained good friends.

It is legendary when referring to Christiaan Barnard's accomplishments that while at the University of Minnesota he could do in a short two-and-a-half years what others needed six or seven years to complete. He obtained a Master of Sciences in Surgery (MS) under Lillehei in 1958 based on studies in the fabrication and testing of a prosthetic aortic valve. The same year, he was awarded a Doctor of Philosophy (PhD) under Professor Wangensteen from studies regarding the etiology of congenital intestinal atresia. This latter work Barnard had started at Cape Town under the leadership of Professor Louw, his eternal mentor and supporter.

When the time at Minnesota came to an end, it was not easy for Barnard to come to this realization and Professor Wangensteen offered to him the possibility of staying on the staff at this prestigious university. Barnard, being a whole-hearted Afrikaaner, followed his heart back to South Africa, returning as initially planned.

By mid-1958, he was in Cape Town again working at Groote Schuur Hospital and developing and organizing the open heart surgery team. They acquired the necessary heart-lung pump from the U.S. government through the mediation of Professor Wangensteen. They needed a chief technician trained on the management of the heart-lung bypass pump, and Carl Goosen filled that position very well. He was initially trained by Barnard on all details of pump operation. Cardiac surgery in the animal surgical laboratory completed the training circle prior to the first human surgery. All had learned the ins and outs of the heart pump, and the beginning of heart surgery at Groote Schuur was in sight!

The heart team began operating on simple and complex cardiac cases with outstanding results. The ability of Barnard and his team was well-demonstrated the world over. In the 1960's after establishing heart surgery at the hospital and community level, Barnard began to organize his efforts regarding the possibility of performing heart transplantation. His excellent plan took him to the U.S., to visit Richmond, Virginia, where he attended the transplant service of David Hume (1917–1973). There he reviewed the technique of heart transplantation with Richard Lower (1929–2008), who had published the pioneering technical paper with Norman Shumway (1923–2006) from California. Barnard also visited Denver, Colorado, where he met Tom Starzl (b.1926) who had been using new and exciting immunosuppressive techniques.[1–5]

Barnard was moving ahead with his well-dreamed plans and the pieces were fitting together perfectly. In the surgical research laboratories he performed heart transplantation in dogs, using all the requirements necessary for human surgery and achieved good results. Furthermore, he transplanted the first kidney in South Africa with particularly good results since the patient lived for many years afterwards.

Everything was ready, then, to proceed with the first human-to-human heart transplant. The recipient had to be selected and the donor had to be found. All things occurred at the right time and Barnard and his team went ahead and realized the first successful human heart transplant at Groote Schuur Hospital, University of Cape Town, South Africa on December 2–3, 1967.[1–5] A very unique and special accomplishment!

For now, let's come back to know better Chris Barnard the man, Chris Barnard the individual, Chris Barnard the human being. We have already mentioned many of his virtues and deficiencies, but let us summarize. In this direction, we can use the opinions of many surgeons who knew him well, as stated in the specially crafted book edited by a cardiac surgeon and student of Barnard's, David Cooper. In *Chris Barnard by Those Who Know Him*, Cooper did an extraordinary job, taking to heart and infinite detail the comments of those who knew Barnard.[11] This book made my job so simple when investigating Barnard's life and accomplishments as seen by his peers and contemporaries.

Many details of Barnard's character and educational goals have been presented previously, but let me concentrate now on those that might be missing. Professor Jannie Louw (1915–1992) met Barnard in 1945 while Chris was in 5th year medical school and Louw was registrar (resident) and in charge of ward and pathology tutorials. Louw remained in contact with Barnard for almost 40 years and probably then knew him better than anyone else. Louw indicated that Chris was hard driven and demonstrated intense "hunger for victory."[11] Louw also said "Chris is an ambitious man but he could also be stubborn and even vindictive."[11] Professor Louw finalized his comments about Barnard's personality and character in the following way:[11]

> "His success was due to his tremendous drive and discipline. He believed that champions must have a "killer instinct" and should be constantly "hungry" to remain at the top. He therefore drove himself to the extreme at all times and did not spare his registrars and nursing staff at the hospital, his assistants in the laboratory, and even his daughter, Deirdre, in her attempts at becoming a water-ski champion."

John Terblanche (b.1935), who eventually became professor and chairman of surgery at the University of Cape Town after Louw, worked under the tutelage of Barnard for many years and at the end went full circle when he became Barnard's chief. Terblanche gives us a clear assessment of the man and the surgeon who was Chris Barnard:[7,11]

> "I first became aware of Chris Barnard in 1957 and 1958 in my latter two years as a medical student at the University of Cape Town. Although student contact was limited he was known as a bright, intelligent young surgeon who had recently returned from a very successful period of postgraduate training in the United States. His few bedside tutorials were excellent and stimulating. I also heard him presenting new data on cardiac physiology to medical and surgical meetings."

Terblanche continued on with his appreciation of Professor Barnard:[7,11]

> "In 1961 I spent a further six months as a clinical registrar in the cardiothoracic department before leaving cardiac surgery to change direction and train as a general surgeon. These were my golden years with Barnard and it was fascinating to be associated with him during this phase of his career. These 18 months gave me considerable insight into the development of Barnard. He was determined to do well. Patients whom he had operated on had to do well. He expected his junior staff to work as long as required and continuously, for days on end, if needed in the interest of his patients."

Terblanche also introduced the Barnard who was impatient, severe and critical when things did not go well in the operating room. "He was a difficult person to work for and his demands were not always reasonable. One felt personally to blame if one of his patients developed a complication or unfortunately died."[7,11]

One can surmise from these recollections that Barnard was a gifted, but at the same time, complex man. He had a strong professional ethic that sometimes did not translate into his personal life. He was moved by intense desire to conquer without consideration for his personal and family well-being. He put others at risk for the great sacrifices he demanded from them. He was a hard-driven man no matter what the cost might be. He was a man of principles who followed only his own direction at all times.

Barnard the Surgeon, the Scientist and Researcher

There is no question that Barnard was a gifted surgeon and an accomplished scientist and researcher. He had the two significant strengths of professional success in a well-rounded academic surgeon, that is clarity of vision as a surgeon and ability to do good scientific research to answer the most critical questions of the profession. Barnard had it all, then. He could operate, achieve good results and perform excellent surgical research that would allow him to take his animal findings to the clinic. Today we call this capability translational research.

Trained as a cardiovascular surgeon and researcher under the auspices of Wangensteen and Lillehei at the recognized Minnesota surgical school, Barnard advanced greatly in applying the principles developed during his American tenure. We have presented his educational developments and now we want to emphasize his surgical expertise and research ability. Again, I will use the words of others who knew him better, since they worked directly with him in the laboratory and the surgical theater. The extracted comments will be shortened to give more opportunities to review Dr. Barnard's stature as surgeon and scientist-researcher.

For his first surgeon chief, professor Louw, Barnard evolved from a good and secure surgeon early on to "an outstanding cardiac surgeon and researcher" as confirmed by international reputation.[11] Professor Terblanche from the same university said, "Barnard was a great clinician and highly competent and innovative surgeon. Many adult and pediatric congenital heart disease cases I assisted him with in 1960 were unique at that time, and his results were outstanding."[11] Lillehei, another of his close teachers while in America, commented on Barnard's surgical ability:[11]

> "I always considered him (Barnard) a reliable technician whom I trusted completely. He was certainly very capable. He probably was not as smooth as Denton Cooley, who is obviously unusual. But as you well know as a surgeon, it's unlikely that anybody, with a few exceptions, is ever born a surgeon — they have to learn. He was a quick learner, there is no doubt about that.... . He was an excellent student.... . He became an excellent technical surgeon through hard work."

I think these examples from his mentors (Louw and Lillehei) and student (Terblanche) give us a fair assessment of Barnard as a surgeon. He was without question a gifted surgeon with an incredible zest for obtaining good results, excellent qualities to expect from someone in the field of surgery!

As a scientist and researcher, Barnard's level of commitment and understanding was very high as well. He frequently formulated research questions, which he often answered through well-planned experimental design. Immediately thereafter, when a response was evident, he applied the answers in the operating room. As I know from my personal experience at Minnesota in surgery and what Barnard possibly learned there, the research process probably was like this: from an initial idea came its development, then the planning in the laboratory with subsequent clinical application. Barnard formulated his complex research questions, processed them, answered them, and applied them in the operating room repeatedly.

I believe that by evaluating his work in the laboratory and the clinic, Barnard was without question an excellent researcher. He was able to pose a great number of questions and, as I said earlier, he utilized the responses on a great number of occasions.

As we move ahead on our quest, we can say that Barnard was a dedicated researcher and scientist since he published 203 papers, as evidenced by the PubMed records, representing a period of 46 years from 1955 to

2001. There were 71 publications prior to the classic paper, *The Operation. A Human Cardiac Transplant*, published in 1967 in the *South African Medical Journal*,[12] and there were 131 articles afterwards. His output certainly was in acceptable numbers compared to other great contributors to the surgical cardiac literature. For example, we reviewed another great heart surgeon pioneer Norman Shumway, this time from the U.S. He had 416 publications listed on PubMed from 1951–2005, a span of 54 years. These publications were obtained in eight more years than Barnard, and with a more elaborate support system at Stanford Cardiothoracic Program, which had a larger staff and more established residency and fellowship programs. Thus, we can say without a doubt that by the sheer number of publications, Barnard made contributions comparable to one of the best American cardiac surgeon pioneers, Norman Shumway.

Barnard the Innovator

A high number of innovations came from the mind and productivity of Christiaan Barnard. We can begin with his initial work on intestinal atresia, which began in South Africa with Professor Louw[8,11] and continued in the U.S. in the laboratories of Professor Wangensteen in Minnesota. Barnard moved from here to Lillehei's laboratories, where he did innovative work on the development and fabrication of an aortic valve, which became his PhD thesis.

Upon his return to Cape Town, Barnard confronted the difficulties with aplomb and intensity, organizing the cardiovascular pump team and all the necessary teachings to begin his heart surgery career in South Africa. He concentrated on cardiac cases. He studied congenital heart anomalies and began treating all of them, from the simple ones like atrial septal defects to complicated cases of tetralogy of Fallot, such as transposition of the great vessels and Ebstein's abnormality. He was highly innovative as he was moving to the top of his field. Barnard was becoming the heart surgeon par excellence in his country and the rest of the world. There was nothing he could not do. He tackled new cases and operations he and others had never performed before. He was innovative, resourceful and ready to accept cases that some other great cardiovascular surgeons could not or would not do. In building his practice, Barnard accepted cases from anywhere. It appeared he was ready to solve any surgical cardiac maladies. His surgical results at the time were beyond those of others in their respective areas. Barnard was ahead of his times then and later on as well, while proceeding toward heart transplantation.

Barnard's innovation continued with the investigation of better ways to design and develop heart valves, like the aortic and the mitral valves, that might require repair. From there he moved to heart transplantation. Surgical techniques, patient management during the operative act, cardiopulmonary pump management and utilizing the best immunosuppressive techniques were all included.

The orthotopic first human-to-human heart transplant occurred in 1967 after full-time preparation by Barnard and his team. Many heart transplants followed and they were performed with equally acceptable skill and success. At some point Barnard's team reached the best results seen in heart transplantation up to that point. In some ways it is disappointing that Barnard did not continue performing orthotopic heart transplants with the same intensity as he did in his early days.[2-5,11]

After orthotopic heart transplants became better accepted and managed in general, Barnard turned his attention to heterotopic heart transplantation in 1973, as a way to offer some extra support for the failing heart. The idea was simple but monumental in scope. The plan was to add a new heart that assisted the poorly working native heart, either as a support for the left ventricle or as biventricular support. Of the 49 consecutive heterotopic heart transplants performed at Cape Town between 1974 and 1983, most were of the biventricular type.[2-5]

In spite of some of the advantages presented by Barnard's group on the use of the heterotopic transplant, this operation did not generate as much outside enthusiasm. Orthotopic heart transplantation remained as the primary indication for irreversible heart failure. Today, it continues to be considered in the same way.

The next interesting idea originating from Barnard's intellectual pursuit was the use of baboon-to-human heart xenotransplantation. In 1977, this event occurred twice, one time being a complete failure and the other time maintaining life for 4 days until the animal heart was rejected and the human heart did not recover.[2-5] These attempts proved, if anything, the incredible thinking and pioneering ability of Barnard and his group, as well as the lack of inhibition in approaching difficult problems. Clearly, Barnard was ahead of his times in many ways.

His innovative approach to surgery and especially to cardiac surgery was well-demonstrated and gave no doubt of the many contributions he made to this field of surgery. His students continued to produce seminal work on hypothermic perfusion storage of the donor heart[2,5] and hormonal replacement therapy for the management of donor stability from the perspective of improved myocardial function.[2,5] The use of thyroid hormones was critical in reaching better organ function after procurement from brain dead donors.

In a nut shell, this is Barnard's work as innovator. He thought of many projects throughout his career and moved ahead by realizing and transferring many of them from the laboratory into the clinical arena. He was an innovator to the core and did not rest until his ideas moved forward. He left the field of cardiac surgery a better place after his retirement in 1983 and his untimely death in 2002.

Barnard's Marital and Family Life

We have previously indicated that from his first marriage with Aletta (Louwtjie) Louw in 1948, two children were born, Deirdre and Andre. Unfortunately, in 1984, when in his early 30's and a beginning pediatric doctor, Andre was found drowning in the bathtub by his wife Gail, who was arriving home from a nursing night call. They had two children together. It was extremely sad and took the whole family by surprise, a very devastating event! In 1969, Barnard's union with Aletta ended in divorce.

The next year, Barnard married Barbara Zoellner, a 19-year-old who gave him two children, Frederick and Christiaan. After 12 years, this second marriage could not continue and divorce occurred in 1982. In spite of Chris' desire to remain married, this was not possible because of his frequent travels and the lack of attention toward his wife and family.

After several years of romantic pursuits, in 1988, Barnard married Karin Setzkorn, who was in her early 20's and more than 40 years younger than him. Together they had two children, Armin-named after a Swiss friend of his, and Lara, possibly named after Dr. Zhivago's wife in the famous Russian novel. In 2000, after 12 years of marriage, Chris and Karin divorced. This time Chris did not marry again.

On September 2, 2001, while vacationing in Cyprus, Barnard, after going for an innocent swim, had a severe asthma attack that took his life. Immediately thereafter the news was spread around the world by the same media who constantly followed him during his life.

Barnard's Financial and Business Considerations

Barnard had made no substantial amount of money and was not interested in it while being a famous heart surgeon in Cape Town. In spite of his international accolades he did not appear to capitalize on them economically. However, near and after his retirement Barnard got involved in several business ventures. One of them was associated with Armin Mattli, owner of the Clinique La Prairie in Switzerland, where the heart pioneer was named director of research and had to support and advertise the use of Glycel cream, which was advertised to prevent aging. Furthermore, Barnard advertised Kellogg's products, Ford Motor Company and the creation of a health center in Cos, Greece-the land of the father of medicine, Hippocrates. He opened restaurants around Cape Town and acquired a ranch as potential sources of income. The noted surgeon was not a businessman and his endeavors did not yield great revenues. His call was not to the business world but to the cardiac surgery arena.

Conclusions and Acknowledgements

Barnard made significant advances in the field of cardiac surgery and performed the first human-to-human heart transplant in the world. His tenacity and dedication took him to places that others could not readily enter. His renowned mentor and surgeon pioneer, C. Walton Lillehei, put it better than others when he said, "I think everybody who knew him in those days was struck by his intense ambition and ability to work — certainly I was....He was very innovative and his research projects bear that out... . He had a prodigious memory... . He accomplished a great deal in enhancing the technical and innovative aspects of surgery."[11] I believe these quotes tell us a great deal about the man and the surgeon. Other aspects of his life have already been included in the text of this work.

In this review and analysis I would like to recognize the incredible amount of work and dedication that David Cooper incorporated into the assessment of Barnard's contributions to heart surgery and the evaluation of his virtues and drawbacks in his professional and personal life.[2,5,11] I am fortunate to have so many writings about Barnard's work and life, which has permitted me to study him in such a great detail.[2–11] Thanks to all of you who have written on Barnard's contributions to medicine, so I could have the luxury of reviewing his life with ample information at hand. The personal writings and books of Barnard have been very helpful as well, when trying to understand the complex man he was.

A note of caution — there are many aspects of the life and accomplishments of Barnard that could not be fully covered in my work, but the excellent references offered in this study can greatly help those interested in pursuing this man and his very much worthwhile biography.

References

1. Toledo-Pereyra LH. (2010) Heart transplantation. *J Invest Surg* **23**:1–5.
2. Cooper DKC. (2001) Christiaan Barnard and his contributions to heart transplantation. *J Heart Lung Transplant* **20**:599–610.
3. Barnard CN, Cooper DKC. (1981) Clinical transplantation of the heart: a review of 13 years' personal experience. *J R Soc Med* **74**:670–674.
4. Reichart BA, Reichenspurner HKC, Odell JA, *et al.* (1987) Heart transplantation at Groote Schuur Hospital, Cape Town. Twenty years' experience. *S Afr Med J* **72**:737–739.
5. Brink JG, Cooper DKC. (2005) Heart transplantation: the contributions of Christiaan Barnard and the University of Cape Town/Groote Schuur Hospital. *World J Surg* **29**:953–961.
6. Rowe DJR. (1979) Dr. Christiaan Barnard: renowned surgeon, egotist but an old-fashioned family doctor at heart. *Can Med Assoc J* **120**:98–99.
7. Terblanche J. (2007) Chris Barnard — a personal tribute to a gifted heart surgeon and a great intellect. *S Afr Med J* **97**:550.
8. Barnard C, Pepper CB. (1970) *One Life*. The MacMillan Co., Toronto. (First American Edition.)

9. Barnard C. (1993) *The Second Life*. Vlaeberg Publishers, Cape Town.

10. Barnard C. (1996) *The Donor*. Michael Joseph Ltd., London.

11. Cooper DKC. (1992) *Chris Barnard — By Those Who Know Him*. Vlaeberg Publishers, Cape Town.

12. Barnard CN. (1967) The operation. A human cardiac transplant: an interim report of a successful operation performed at Groote Schuur Hospital, Cape Town. *S Afr Med J* **41**:1271–1274.

16

Heart Transplantation

by Luis H. Toledo-Pereyra, MD, PhD

Dedication

> *The courage and commitment of*
> *Louis Washkansky and the Darvall*
> *family as well as the innovative spirit*
> *and determination of Christiaan*
> *Barnard and his team are especially*
> *commended and recognized.*

That heart transplantation became a reality is still hard to conceive![1-15] The sole fact of being able to remove a normal heart from a deceased individual, excising the bad heart from a patient with irreversible heart disease and then implanting the donor heart into a living patient was once part of imaginative science fiction, an unthinkable dream, one we were unlikely to see in our life time.

Nevertheless, a series of important events occurred, springing from hard work and the innovative spirit of a great number of individuals, culminating in the extraordinary case performed in the winter of 1967 at Groote Schuur Hospital in South Africa. The genius of Christiaan Barnard (1922–2002) was the intellectual and decisive force behind these pioneering events. Our intention is to comment on some of the various historical

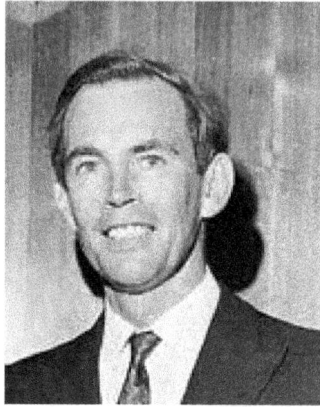

Figure 16.1.   Christiaan N. Barnard (1922–2002) in 1968 photo.

aspects surrounding the study of the heart and those related to heart transplantation and to review some philosophical and ethical concepts pertaining to this incredible development.

Long Before Cape Town, South Africa

Long before that historic transplantation in Cape Town, South Africa, other discoverers had begun their quest for defining the heart's anatomy and function in cities as far flung as Padua, London and Bologna. Stretching back into antiquity, physicians in Stagira, Alexandria, Pergamon, Persia, Egypt and other locations were interested in the heart as well.[1,2] They sought an understanding of anatomy, physiology and some vital characteristics regarding the heart and its vascular components. The heart occupied the center of attention from the beginning of history. The heart represented the center of imagination. Physicians and philosophers dissected the heart intellectually and considered it to be a vital spirit. The heart was the critical piece and the central element in the circulation of the blood. Medical philosophers utilized the heart to demonstrate kindness, understanding, life, death and a spectrum of emotional responses.

Aristotle (384–322 BC) from Stagira viewed the heart as the guiding torch of human and animal function; he "identified the heart as the most important organ of the body and the first to form according to his observations on the chick embryo."[1,15] Years after Aristotle, other Greek surgeon-anatomists and physiologists such as Herophilus and Erasistratus, while in Alexandria, refuted Aristotle's claim, maintaining that the brain and not the heart was the primary organ of the economy.[1,2,15] Centuries later, Galen (129–199 AD) of Pergamon arrived to support Aristotle's point of view and shed some light on the role of the heart by saying, "The heart is the root of all faculties and….the veins connected the operations of the liver to the heart which circulated vital spirits throughout the body via the arteries."[1,2,15]

In spite of the views expressed at the Alexandrian School of Anatomy, the heart continued to be perceived as the center of the human economy. During the Middle Ages, the Persian master Avicenna (981–1032 AD) took the position of Aristotle, and thus Galen, and considered that the heart "was an intelligent organ that controlled and directed all others."[1,15] Two centuries later, the Syrian/Egyptian physician Ibn al-Nafis (1213–1288 AD) concentrated on the pulmonary and capillary circulation and no particular attention was given to the heart.[1] Only during the Renaissance did physicians come back to attend to matters of the heart.

En Route to Cape Town Through the Renaissance and Beyond

Cape Town was still in the distant future, but the first steps for characterizing the heart were being taken. Great physicians and scientists were attempting to define the heart and the circulation. Previous civilizations had reported on the heart but the Greeks had made their own excellent contributions to understanding the heart, principally through Aristotle, Herophilus, Erasistratus and Galen. During the Renaissance, physicians challenged Galen but not Aristotle regarding the view of the heart and the circulation of blood, not knowing that both of them held many similar ideas since Galen had followed Aristotle's cardiovascular observations. During the 15th, 16th and early 17th centuries, Leonardo da Vinci, Andreas Vesalius, Miguel Servetus, Realdo Columbus, Andreas Caesalpinus and Hieronymus Fabricius made their own significant contributions to the recognition of the four chambers of the heart, the lack of septum communications between the two ventricles, the confirmation of the pulmonary circulation and the existence of valves in the venous system. All of these findings would support and enlighten William Harvey (1578–1657) on his circulatory theory.[1,15]

Keep in mind that without all the knowledge exposed by these early pioneers, Barnard would have found the road to that first heart transplant in Cape Town in 1967 extremely difficult! A key development necessary for success in South Africa was Harvey's immensely important circulatory theory describing the movement of the blood. He published his ideas and experimental findings in 1628 and the world soon realized that the blood had a circular movement, that the arteries carried the blood out and that the veins, through the function of their own valves, returned blood to the heart, that the heart had its own motion and that it contracted and expelled the blood. Of course, this great scientific discovery recognized the importance of valves and other critical details.

After the Renaissance, Marcello Malpighi (1628–1694), Richard Lower (1631–1691) and Antony van Leeuwenhoek (1632–1723) contributed critical elements to the discovery and affirmation of other aspects of the circulatory system. For instance, Malpighi introduced the presence of capillaries in the blood system, Lower experimented with the circulation and transfusion of blood from animal to animal and from animal to human, and Leeuwenhoek observed many blood vessels and studied them carefully. These three scientists completed their observations shortly before and after Harvey's time.[1,14]

18th Century Medical Contributions to Cape Town

Cape Town remained distant during the 18th century, although the anatomy of the heart was better understood, particularly with new work introduced in 1706 by French physician Raymond de Vieussens (1635–1715), who studied the heart and circulation in health and disease. Years later, in 1733, the English physiologist Stephen Hales (1677–1761) showed the feasibility of measuring the blood pressure in animals and a few years afterwards the Italian anatomist and first modern pathologist, Giovanni Battista Morgagni (1682–1771), introduced the value of pathological anatomy in clinical disease in 1761. In the same year, Austrian physician Leopold Auenbrugger (1722–1809) demonstrated the importance of percussion around the heart, allowing clinicians to determine the size of the heart by percussion.[14]

From earlier studies of well-admired teachers like the English physician Thomas Sydenham (1624–1689), the Dutch clinician Herman Boerhaave (1668–1738), as well as the Scottish medical master William Cullen (1710–1790), the importance of clinical findings in the diagnosis of heart disease was carefully integrated. These outstanding clinicians opened the doors to recognizing disease clinically, and started to consolidate symptoms and signs into syndromes and well-established clinical entities.[5,6,15] Progress was being made towards identifying heart disease.

Reaching Cape Town by Advancing into 19th and 20th Century Medicine and Surgery

In 1816, the French physician Rene T. H. Laennec (1781–1826) invented the stethoscope, in 1846 ether anesthesia was successfully utilized by American Surgeon-in-Chief John Collins Warren (1778–1856) at Massachusetts General Hospital, and in 1865 the antiseptic method was introduced by English Master Surgeon Joseph Lister (1827–1912). Prior to the end of the 19th century, in 1896, William Roentgen (1845–1923) occupied the attention of the world with the discovery of X-rays, which had a positive effect in examining the heart and surrounding structures as well. All these needed changes were critical stops on the road to the heart transplant in Cape Town. However, many more advances were required and they appeared as the 20th century commenced.

In 1903, the Dutch physician and physiologist Willem Einthoven (1860–1927) invented the electrocardiograph, and in 1912 the American doctor James B. Herrick (1861–1954) described heart disease resulting from arteriosclerotic damage in a more specific manner. He reported on the mechanism of myocardial infarction due to thrombosis of the coronary arteries.[14] In 1929, German surgeon Dr. Werner Forssmann (1904–1979) had the audacity to perform successful human cardiac catheterization on himself. Twelve years later, in 1941, the Frenchman Andre F. Cournand (1895–1988) and the American Dickinson W. Richards (1895–1973), working at Columbia in New York, introduced the use of cardiac catheterization as a diagnostic tool, and in 1958 the American doctor

F. Mason Sones (1918–1985) introduced diagnostic coronary angiography.[14] These significant contributions opened the wide field of cardiovascular pathology and diagnostic science that permitted Barnard to reach the outskirts of Cape Town.

Cardiac Surgery at Minnesota Before Cape Town

In 1952, F. John Lewis (1916–1993) performed the first successful open heart surgery under hypothermia at the University of Minnesota. This case permitted others to consider cardiac surgery as a possibility. The details for clinical open heart surgery had not been worked out and only simple cases with short repairs could be performed with the Lewis technique. Two years later, in 1954, C. Walton Lillehei (1918–1998) and his group at the University of Minnesota completely changed the field of cardiac surgery. Indeed, they revolutionized this surgical arena when open heart surgery was successfully performed with crossed circulation.[12] Many congenital heart defects were fully repaired with outstanding results given the state of the art at the time. Open heart surgery had been unleashed and possibilities for fixing all types of cardiac pathology existed from this point on! More developments occurred during this period and great cardiac surgical pioneers filled the halls of operating rooms around the world.

In 1956, Barnard came to Minnesota for a two-year fellowship under Professor Owen Wangensteen (1898–1981), chairman of the department of surgery, and C. Walton Lillehei, cardiac surgical star at the university, and Richard Varco (1912–2004), a notable senior surgeon in the program. These two years were exciting for Barnard, who worked intensely, learned as much as he could, operated in the animal laboratory and, whenever possible, in the clinic. He was committed to taking as much as he could from this program, which at the time was the center of cardiac surgery in the world!

Barnard knew he had seen and done all he could in cardiac surgery at Minnesota and was ready to take everything to Cape Town. The contributions included a cardiac pump and an oxygenator, graciously negotiated by Dr. Wangensteen and installed by the U.S. government in the newly created South African cardiac program. Barnard was well on his way to achieving his goal of cardiac transplantation when he departed for Groote Schuur Hospital in Cape Town.

Into Cape Town Towards Groote Schuur Hospital

Chris, as his friends referred to him, returned from America, where he had learned all the do's and don'ts associated with cardiac surgery, and was ready to operate on human hearts with a very distant view of heart transplantation at Groote Schuur Hospital still on the horizon. There was no reason to wait in taking the first steps toward successful transplantation.

First, Barnard set up an experimental surgical cardiac program where he could review the surgical techniques learned at Minnesota; second, he moved into the clinical arena tackling simple first and then complicated congenital cardiac defects; third, he developed a surgical intensive care unit second to none for the care of his patients; fourth, he began to incorporate his own ideas into developing innovative surgical techniques, prosthetic valves and so on.[8,9]

By the early 1960's, Barnard was well-established in Cape Town at Groote Schuur Hospital. He was in charge of the cardiac program and all surgical research endeavors at Groote Schuur. He was the most advanced cardiac surgeon in Africa, and one of the leading surgeons in correcting congenital defects in the world. Barnard had advanced to a position of knowledge, respect and attention that permitted him to explore other endeavors, both new and progressive.

Barnard Enters the Heart Transplant Preparation Phase

As Barnard began thinking more seriously about the possibility of embarking into heart transplantation, he knew he had to return to the United States where he would learn immunosuppressive techniques, review the Lower and Shumway surgical procedure for experimental heart transplantation, and reinforce his possible approach to the transplantation of the heart. In 1967, before the first heart transplant operation in Cape Town, he visited David Hume in Virginia for three months, Tom Starzl in Colorado for two weeks, and while in Virginia he observed Richard Lower performing a canine heart transplant with his newly introduced technique in association with Norman Shumway.[8,9] With this experience under his belt, Barnard returned to South Africa to make arrangements for a potential human heart transplant.

Back in Cape Town, before the heart transplant operation, Barnard performed a clinical kidney transplant to gain access to the best immuno-suppressive therapy available at the time. His results with one patient proved to be a complete success. Now, he had applied immunosupression, he had studied all immunological techniques utilized in America and personally used them in Cape Town. In addition, according to John Terblanche, one of his students, Barnard performed many transplant operations on dogs.[13] He was ready, then, to start the human experiment!

December 3, 1967 — Heart Transplant Arrives

No one in the world had performed a heart orthotopic-human-to-human transplant. No one yet possessed the audacity. No one was willing to be the first, particularly after the failed and highly criticized heart xenotransplant (chimpanzee to human) performed in 1964 by James Hardy in Mississippi.[8,9] Without the world really knowing, one person in this distant place on the planet was preparing his team to proceed with the operation, perhaps the biggest surgical advance in the world! What was about to be attempted at Groote Schuur had amazing implications. Once the heart had been taken from the donor, there was no turning back.

Barnard identified a recipient in Louis Washkansky, a 53-year-old man suffering from innumerable diseases, including coronary insufficiency, diabetes, peripheral vascular disease, and with a history of smoking. In addition, massive edema uncontrollable by regular measures complicated the recipient's clinical picture. Washkansky was by no means the best available recipient then and would probably be considered very high risk today.[8,9]

The donor represented the other side of the equation, being equally as important as the recipient. Because of the South African policy of apartheid, Barnard felt that a white donor was important to diminish potential criticism by the enemies of the country. In this way, when Denise Darvall, a 23-year-old white woman and victim of a car accident became brain-dead, the heart-donor team moved ahead with the procurement of her heart. Barnard also felt that a physician examiner should pronounce the patient dead, since his belief was that the "patient was not dead until the doctor said so."[8,9]

Darvall's heart was removed by Barnard's assistants. The recipient was prepared in an adjacent room by Barnard himself, who took the diseased heart out and placed the new heart in. The immensity of this procedure had no comparison to previous surgical procedures he had performed. This was a unique event, difficult to compare to any other procedure, since there was no precedence in this case.

The operation went well and Mr. Washkansky fully recovered, enjoying a full life for at least 12 days before his health began to deteriorate. He developed pneumonia and later septicemia, from which he died on the 18th postoperative day. The details of his medical management and the use of anti-rejection drugs are not the purpose of this work, which emphasizes the origins of clinical heart transplantation. In a similar manner, subsequent heart transplants will not be discussed, as we are focusing on the first transplant performed in the Barnard's long series of transplants. Suffice it to say that his second heart transplant patient, Philip Blaiberg, lived for 19 months and thus gave hope to the thousands of patients who would become potential candidates for heart transplantation.

Cape Town, Groote Schuur Hospital, Christiaan Barnard and Heart Transplantation: Concluding Remarks

There are no words to describe the incredible odyssey of clinical heart transplantation. Cape Town, Groote Schuur Hospital and Christiaan Barnard came together at a particular time in history to successfully amalgamate the best of all three. Without this symbiotic relationship, the full experiment of heart transplantation might never have occurred. Barnard was the essential element uniting all the various phases of this experiment. He came at the right time to Cape Town, attended Groote Schuur Hospital for his initial surgical training and proceeded to Minnesota, where he received his education in cardiovascular surgery and was part of the large and exciting Minnesota experiment. I would even suggest that without the opportunity that Barnard had at the University of Minnesota, realizing his dreams would have been practically impossible. Minnesota permitted him to see, taste and be part of a unique surgical cardiovascular team led by Lillehei and Varco, with the support of the well-known chief of the surgical department, Wangensteen.

The progress of history from antiquity to 1967, when the first human heart transplant was performed, has been briefly considered and should serve as an example for future generations of leaders in surgery and medicine.

Before we close, it is important to recognize the vision, fortitude, impetus, desire and commitment of one man, Christiaan Neethling Barnard, who because of his innovative spirit made clinical heart transplantation a reality. Doctor Barnard should be considered in this sense the "Father of Heart Transplantation."

Personal Acknowledgement

I would like to pay recognition to Barnard's South African cardiac surgery group for the excellent publications they have put forward and in particular the superb works published by D.K.C. Cooper. Their academic output has been a significant part of my publication. Without their input I would not have been able to complete this paper.

References

1. Graubard M. (1964) *Circulation and Respiration. The Evolution of an Idea.* Harcourt, Brace and World, Inc., New York and Burlingame.
2. Singer C. (1957) *Short A History of Anatomy and Physiology from the Greeks to Harvey.* Dover Publications Inc., New York.
3. Toledo-Pereyra LH. (2005) *Vignettes on Surgery, History and Humanities.* Landes Bioscience, Austin, Texas.
4. Toledo-Pereyra LH. (2007) *Origins of the Knife. The Encounters with the History of Surgery.* Landes Bioscience, Georgetown, Texas.
5. History of Medicine. From wikipedia.org. Accessed January 15, 2010.
6. History of Surgery. From wikipedia.org. Accessed January 20, 2010.
7. Barnard CN. (1981) Clinical transplantation of the heart: a review of 13 years' personal experience. *J R Soc Med* **74**:670–674.
8. Cooper DKC. (2001) Christiaan Barnard and his contributions to heart transplantation. *J Heart Lung Transplant* **20**:599–610.
9. Brink JG, Cooper DKC. (2005) Heart transplantation. The contributions of Christiaan Barnard and the university of Cape Town/Groote Schuur hospital. *World J Surg* **29**:953–961.

10. Barnard CN. (1967) The operation: a human cardiac transplant: an interim report of a successful operation at Groote Schuur Hospital, Cape Town. *S Afr Med J* **41**:1271–1274.
11. Hunt SA, Haddad F. (2008) The changing face of heart transplantation. *J Am Coll Cardiol* **52**:587–598.
12. Cut to the heart. Pioneers of heart surgery. Nova online. From www.pbs.org.
13. Terblanche J. (2007) Chris Barnard — a personal tribute to a gifted heart surgeon and a great intellect. *S Afr Med J* **97**:550.
14. Individual names of various scientific and medical contributors to this story have been researched through the internet including sources like Pubmed, Medline, Wikipedia and Google.
15. History of the heart. From www.stanford.edu/class/history13/. Accessed January 29, 2010.

Art, Surgery and Transplantation

by Luis H. Toledo-Pereyra, MD, PhD

Introduction

In 1996, well-known transplant pioneer Roy Calne (b. 1930) published a book called *Art, Surgery and Transplantation*. In it he conveyed his passion for art, his knowledge and practice of transplantation and his own artistic impression of his patients and the specialty overall. He handsomely succeeded and was able to capably represent the humanistic side of surgery.[1]

The important question for this essay concerns how to better perceive and study the work of Calne contained in his book. After all, transplantation is, like surgery, both an art and a science. It is clear that we need to understand what Calne was trying to represent in his elegant book and how we could receive his message through his paintings and writings.

Our intention here goes to the fundamental analysis of the important work of Calne as it pertains to the interaction of art, surgery and transplantation. In addition, we proceed beyond his art and embark on a brief review of art and surgery as they relate to the evolution of both disciplines through history. We begin chronologically and conclude with the unique work of Calne.

Initial Stages in Art and Surgery

Art and surgery have been constantly intertwined. Surgery is an art on its own and can be readily excelled at when the artistic expression is expanded under usual conditions. Surgery is also a science and is represented by the knowledge and limitations of the surgeon-scientist. When both are combined we can easily visualize the potentials of this strong arm of medicine.

The first attempts at manifesting the art of surgery came in the caves of Lascaux where bison were seen with protruding intestines after arrows injured the abdominal wall. These paintings depict occurrences that happened thousands of years ago, and the depictions were unique developments at the time!

In the historic era, Egyptian artists painted circumcisions. They expressed and elevated the importance of this form of surgical treatment through art. Other artistic events were limited in scope and significance until Leonardo da Vinci (1452–1519) produced his well-recognized anatomical art. Leonardo captured the imagination of the medical and surgical world by illustrating anatomy in a way never seen before. He carefully drew details of bones, muscles, joints, organs, arteries, veins, nerves and other structures. However, Leonardo's artistic anatomical expression was not actually available until the 19th century when his drawings were discovered in an abandoned trunk in an English castle. Because of this, we have considered Leonardo as the "Hidden Father of Modern Anatomy" due to his advanced understanding of the human body and to having created the first elaborate anatomical drawings. This work, however, was not uncovered until after the work of Vesalius had been published.[2]

Andreas Vesalius (1514–1564) shocked the medical and surgical world by introducing the best jewel of anatomical books, *De Humani Corporis Fabrica,* in 1543. Before that time nothing equal had been considered. Remember that the works of Leonardo had been inadvertently hidden until the 19th century.[2]

Leaving aside the important aspects of the accuracy of the anatomical depictions in Vesalius' book, the art reflected in those pictures was monumental.[3] It is by now certain that the artist or artists who worked on the anatomical drawings of *De Humani Corporis Fabrica* were from the school of Titian, and it is assumed that one of them was Stephan van Calcar. (1499–1546?)

Whoever was responsible, the reality is that those works were extraordinary artistic expressions, clearly the best since they attended to both the science and the art of surgery. Finally the surgeons of the time had something they could use during their scientific inquiries.

Vesalius' book was so well presented that everyone could easily understand whatever was necessary for the anatomist and surgeon to advance the field to a higher level. Art and surgery were close companions in the maturation of medicine.

Rembrandt and His Anatomy Lessons

Rembrandt H. van Rijn (1606–1669) was a young painter when he took up the art of surgery by painting "The Anatomy Lesson of Dr. Nicolaes Tulp" (1632). Twenty-four years later and now as a mature painter who was considered a genius, he executed "The Anatomy Lesson of Dr. Joan Deijman" (1656). Both of these superb works occupied the attention of artists and surgeons at the time.

Rembrandt's art was clear, well-defined, with Caravaggio's intense dark colors, and attending to the details of the anatomical and surgical figure. Rembrandt emphasized not only anatomy but clinical function as well. In "The Anatomy Lesson of Dr. Tulp" he traced the figure at many levels, advancing the progression of the clinical response to tendon injury on the forearm and centering his attention on the individual body.

Rembrandt reflected high Renaissance times by attending to anatomy as the defining element of medicine and surgery. There was no question that Rembrandt followed the trends of his era when nothing was more important than the human figure. As other developments occurred, artists consistently refined the art of anatomy and the art of medicine.

Roy Calne accurately explained the art and medicine of the Renaissance by indicating:

"The coming together of art and medicine in the Renaissance was a necessary step towards the liberation of both subjects, from the previous conventions and restrictions imposed by the church and society. During this period, many outstanding works of art were commissioned and were displayed in numerous public buildings. Scientific observation and experiment yielded tremendous results, one being the understanding of anatomy and physiology. It was only with this essential knowledge that reliable and effective treatments for disease and injury could be developed."[1]

Modern Art and Surgery

Once anatomy was well accepted and physiology came under more scrutiny, surgery was better defined within the confines of art. In the mid-19th century, art was being directed at the specific operations that surgeons were utilizing in the treatment of disease. Art and surgery were equally contributing to their respective benefits. Surgeons and artists were working together to recognize the inners workings of the human structure. The surgeon needed to repair the injury or excise the damage and the artist needed to conceive the best form to draw the anatomical elements for surgical purposes.

After Vesalius and van Calcar, books of anatomy opened a great opportunity for artists to draw the minute details of the human body. In the 19th century, the works of Gray, Testut, Cunningham and many others in various countries portrayed in exquisite detail the analytical forms of anatomy. As far as anatomy was concerned, art and surgery went hand-in-hand to express the benefits of the anatomical conception. Surgeons used art and anatomy to the benefits of their surgery and the patients they were curing.

Modern art has been more encompassing in its expression of form. Even though drawing was critical to the figure, it took a dramatic leap from the Renaissance expression. For modern artists, it was possible to enter approximations and conceive, in many instances, a more relaxed presentation. It was accepted in this way that art could be understood in all its forms. Surgery took those manifestations and incorporated them into its main work. Art and surgery were becoming frequently accepted partners.

The pure work of anatomy and surgical techniques, by definition, do not change much. However, one change has come from the additional precision and knowledge in drawing beyond the skin. Whether the anatomical drawing was perfect or not, surgeons rely on their representation according to accepted techniques of the times. Surgeons wanted to know what lay beneath and how they could solve their surgical technical problems.

Many years later, great surgeon artists like Harvey Cushing (1865–1937) would draw in the operating room and utilize the drawings in the conception and development of treatments. Cushing was completely committed to enhancing anatomical figures and to the realization that neurosurgical events could be better understood if one would specify details with drawing and artistic expression.

More of Modern Art

When we carefully examine the 19th century, and particularly the later part of it, the Philadelphia artist Thomas Eakins (1844–1916) occupied a place of honor in both art and surgery. Two particular pieces conquered the attention of those who had the opportunity to admire them in minute detail. The first, "The Gross Clinic" (1875), captivated the attention of the medical and artistic world as far as the realistic presentation of the surgeon's operating conditions at the time. Samuel D. Gross (1805–1884), one of the most distinguished American professors of surgery of his epoch, was performing the surgery, which consisted a debridement of the bones of the leg instead of the typical amputation performed as a regular treatment at the time. The backdrop is the Thomas Jefferson University operating room.

Fourteen years later, in 1889, Eakins painted "The Agnew Clinic," a superb surgical painting of a breast surgery case performed by the noted University of Pennsylvania professor of surgery, David H. Agnew (1818–1892). The Agnew painting demonstrates the antiseptic techniques that had been accepted after the earlier painting. The surgeon, assistants and operating room nurse are wearing white clothing and the operating room is impeccably clean. Both of these works were criticized at the time but were later acclaimed by the scientific and artistic community.[4]

Even though many other art works have appeared since Eakins, very few reached the level of excellence seen in the canvases introduced by the recognized Philadelphia painter. "The Night of San Juan: Field Hospital" (1898), an ink wash on paper by William Glacken (1870–1938), the "Base Hospital" (1918) a lithograph by George Bellows (1882–1925), the excellent photographic work by Max Thorek (1880–1960), the "Front Line Surgery" (1943) a painting by John Steuart Curry (1897–1946), and the

"Babcock Surgical Clinic" (1944–1945) a painting by Furman J. Finck (1900–1997) are just a few examples of the extraordinary works produced more recently.

Back to Roy Calne's Artistic Work: *Art, Surgery and Transplantation*

Roy Calne gives credit to the renowned Scottish painter John Bellany (b. 1942) as the one who started him "on the road to painting the story of transplantation."[1] In *Art, Surgery and Transplantation*, the transplant surgeon-artist introduces several paintings by Bellany, produced when he was recovering from liver transplantation performed by Calne in 1988. Consequently, artist and surgeon established a close bond because of this unique circumstance. Calne took the advice of Bellany and accomplished a great number of outstanding paintings showing the art of surgical transplantation.

Peter Morris, the former Oxford Nuffield Professor of Surgery and master transplant surgeon himself, indicated that professor Calne "attempted to depict the association between painting and illness, with particular emphasis on the surgeon's role in the management of disease." Morris continued by saying that Calne recorded on canvas his patients, the surgical operations and the most significant events of the curative process.[1]

In the first Foreword of Calne's book, Mary Lou and Tony Monaco, well-known wife and transplant surgeon-husband, dear friends of Roy Calne, defined art, surgery and transplantation through the paintings of the surgeon artist, but in addition they handsomely reviewed the history of this endeavor by going back to other surgeon and medical artists such as Joseph Wilder, Henry Tonks and Richard Stark. They ended with Thomas Eakins, identifying him as the master painter of art and surgery.[1] They further added that "such art (Eakins) makes a marvelous contribution to the cultural lives of people and can never be dismissed."[1] Furthermore, they accurately said, "each work of art makes a statement about the period of history in which it was painted and brings aesthetic and emotional pleasure to many people."[1]

Roy Calne accumulated a large body of unique paintings, including those of transplant surgeons and physicians, transplant patients, and many of the incredible details associated with those individuals and the transplant surgical events. For the first time, Calne brought attention to the relationship between art and surgical transplantation. He dissected the discipline in a manner never seen before. Through art, he amplified the understanding of the specter of pain in the evolution of the disease of the transplanted patient, he revealed the anatomical characteristics of transplanted organs, he advanced the identification and comprehension of the "moments of truth" in the operating room and he enhanced the better perception and analysis of potential transplant complications.

A Personal Note

I have known Roy Calne for many years, possibly since 1973, and have been impressed with his science and contributions to surgical transplantation. What I did not know was his prowess in the art associated with transplantation. It was not until I acquired his outstanding book *Art, Surgery and Transplantation* in 1996 that his art greatly touched many aspects of my own knowledge and contribution to transplantation.

Two years after Calne's book was published, in 1998, when our transplant program at Borgess Medical Center, affiliated with Michigan State University in Kalamazoo, was temporarily closed, I began taking art lessons, concentrating on painting at the Kalamazoo Institute of Arts. That experience helped me better understand and appreciate Calne's special book. In making my own art, especially painting, I realized what Calne had done. He had made a very special and unique contribution to the art and science of transplantation.

In reviewing Calne's book and remembering my many years in surgical transplantation, I cannot but feel excited about all those special moments of my life. The book of Roy Calne brings back many special memories. For instance, I recall many personalities and events that are still fresh, such as the figure of my good friend and advisor Felix Rapaport, the memories of my conversations with Tom Starzl, the times of discussion with my Mexican friend and colleague Rafael Valdez, the preservation transplant pioneer Fred Belzer, the remembrances of an afternoon with Norman Shumway in Kalamazoo, where his parents are buried, the good manners of Paul Terasaki and Bill Wall, the accomplishments of Rene Kuss and Joseph Murray, the contributions of Tony Monaco, Peter Morris,

Maurice Slapak, H.M. Lee, Fritz Bach and Jon van Rood, to mention many of the distinguished transplant personalities who were captured by the magic brush of professor Roy Calne.

I particularly enjoyed Calnes's chapter "The Urge to Paint." Fresh and well-presented, it told in a few pages the story of Calne's evolution as a painter. Art was practically another life on its own,[1] a very impressive enterprise and not an easy task under any conditions! Calne learned graphic art and painting early, moved into learning from the classics, and advanced later to Chinese painting by learning from Singapore surgeon Earl Lu. The Scottish master John Bellany taught Calne the principles of figurative painting. Calne, at every step, advanced his art and moved in many directions, each helping and securing his own style. With all these advances, Calne dominated painting in a way that was comparable to many artists of his generation.

Conclusion

The work of Calne has filled a significant vacuum, especially in regards to the art of transplantation, pioneers, patients, events, and surgical moments. His work shows a new way to represent the field and exert a new influence regarding the best way to treat a transplant patient humanely. Art embodies not only aesthetics, but becomes information and therapy for patient and surgeon alike.

References

1. Calne R. (1996) *Art, Surgery and Transplantation.* Williams and Wilkins Europe, Ltd., London.
2. Toledo-Pereyra LH. (2005) Leonardo da Vinci. In: LH Toledo-Pereyra (ed.). *Vignettes on Surgery, History and Humanities.* Landes Biosciences, Georgetown, Texas, pp. 38–40.
3. Sherzoi H. (2005) Andreas Vesalius. In: LH Toledo-Pereyra (ed.). *Vignettes on Surgery, History and Humanities.* Landes Biosciences, Georgetown, Texas, pp. 44–45.
4. Toledo-Pereyra LH. (1998) Thomas Eakins. In: LH Toledo-Pereyra (ed.). *Historia, Cirugia y Cultura.* Editorial Ciencia y Cultura Latino Americana, Mexico, pp. 139–152.

18

Believing in Yourself

by Luis H. Toledo-Pereyra, MD, PhD

What if I told you that believing in yourself is the most important characteristic in your evolving life and career? That is absolutely true, I think. Let me explain as I apply this assertion to the surgeon's way of living and professional goals.

Statement of the Problem

It is apparently well known, or rather implicitly understood, that surgeons are supposed to be so sure of themselves that they cannot exude anything but confidence. It is also assumed that surgeons trust their decisions so much that the opportunity for error is not even considered. These two statements are not necessarily correct and are part of a commonly stereotyped behaviour frequently used to define practicing surgeons. Specialists and surgeons-in-training can acknowledge the stereotype but should also exert the effort to portray themselves and their profession more realistically and positively.

The Issue of Believing in Yourself

Exuberant confidence and poorly understood trust are not desirable traits for surgeons who believe in themselves. Believing in yourself is accepting what is good and what is bad or incomplete about yourself or your professional activity. Believing in yourself is realistically viewing your deficiencies and your willingness to improve with dedicated effort. Believing in yourself is patting yourself on the back when you notice good results or have helped a fellow human being. Believing in yourself is not being afraid of accepting that you are good, that you can help patients, and that you can make life more livable for them and their families. Believing in yourself is honestly and bravely attending to the needs of your patients with the confidence of someone who knows the field, has reviewed the pathology many times, and has effectively intervened in many similar situations.

Believing in Yourself makes you a Better Surgeon and Better Human Being

For the surgical resident or surgical Fellow-in-training or someone who has just finished the educational years of commitment to surgery, believing in yourself becomes a particularly essential attitude.

If you are like me and many residents and fellows, you may at times have lost your surgical identity for a variety of reasons. Without being fully inclusive, the reasons can relate to following faculty directions at all times, as well as to being subjected, in the name of education, to not infrequent downgrading of your surgical abilities while you were attempting to master certain complex procedures. Even though this training approach is changing, on some occasions the change is not fast enough.

Under all circumstances, the surgical trainee or recently graduated surgeon needs to be and remain resilient. In trying times, believing in yourself becomes or should become an essential component of your surgical life. Let me address this issue in more detail, since believing in yourself makes you a better surgeon and better human being.

How do you Reach the State of Believing in Yourself?

Of course, believing in yourself is not a task accomplished in a few hours, but rather a prolonged, committed exercise in re-emphasizing to yourself the positive values of knowledge, experience, and attention to detail that you possess. Build upon these characteristics and convey to yourself these facts — that you can certainly do the surgical operation since you have done it before, that you have knowledge since you have studied this particular topic many times, and that you will pay attention to details since you will observe and avoid possible complications, and thus remain before all else a safe and competent surgeon.

Now, let us talk about specific means to reach the state of believing in yourself: (1) Know the topic theoretically; (2) Strategize the operative procedure in your mind, or better yet, in writing with specific steps to save time and prevent complications; (3) Know the complications and how to get out of trouble; (4) Do not rush through the surgical procedure but take your time and operate at the pace that fits you since safety is very important; and (5) Follow your patient closely. If all these steps are covered, you are a surgeon who will and should believe in him or herself, because you are, and believe it, an excellent surgeon.

Is Believing in Yourself Really Necessary?

I certainly think so. Believing in yourself represents a positive and forward attitude of the surgical trainee or practicing surgeon. Creating or cultivating this attitude would give the surgical professional the emotional basis for enjoying this chosen field of medicine and for reaching superior levels of practice.

Believing in yourself is uplifting for any professional discipline and, indeed, for any human endeavor. It is very plausible to think that professionals who trust and believe in themselves have more opportunities to succeed in life.

Advancing your particular choice of surgical or medical practice possesses a clearer outlook if you believe in what you do and represent. Believing in yourself will give you an added benefit when considering the possibility of participating in the advances of medicine or surgery.

Does History Support the Concept of Believing in Yourself?

As far as I can determine, history has been generous with those who believe in themselves. In fact, history might be saying to us, "Believe in yourself and you will be able to help your patients better and perhaps to advance the surgical sciences to heights never seen before."

Examples of surgeons who believed in themselves are numerous. From surgeons of antiquity like Galen (129–200),[1] to those of modern times like Blalock (1899–1964),[2] Wangensteen (1898–1981),[3] Lillehei (1918–1999)[4] and others,[5] they showed us their firm desire to believe in themselves, their works and their lives. This is not to say that they experienced no disappointments during their professional practice. In fact, intervening with new treatments was a source of major concern for all of them. See, for instance, how Galen was unable to cure a great number of his patients in the gladiators' arena, how Blalock did not reach complete heart repair for blue babies, how Wangensteen was remiss in offering an effective cure for peptic ulcer disease, and how Lillehei in all his wisdom did not foresee the development of heart transplantation. Many other similar considerations could be offered for other surgical professionals.

Truthfully, the previous examples give us the opportunity to reflect upon the deeds of these great individuals and upon their imperfections too, how they struggled to find good treatments, how failure was not far away in some instances, and most of all, on the reality that these pioneering surgeons at no point stopped believing in themselves. In the same manner, I would like to think we can reach out and remain firm believers in ourselves and our extraordinary possibilities. Let us try together. I believe we can do it and that we can make this an uplifting endeavor!

Other Examples in Daily Practice

On more than a few occasions during my surgical career, I and others have encountered perplexing surgical operating situations that have required reaching down to the depths of surgical knowledge and experience and, more importantly, to the depths of character and mental toughness. Not infrequently, determination and believing in yourself represent the saving grace in these sometimes desperate and sometimes routine situations.

The question is how can we better prepare ourselves for this kind of development? The most likely answer is that there is no well-structured plan that can be followed for the difficult cases that challenge you and me to the core of our surgical genes. My only advice is that if we persist in believing in ourselves, that if we believe we can do these complicated or even sometimes innocent, but unusual cases, I know we can be successful. The main ingredient, then, would be to believe in yourself at all times. Believe me!

I am fully aware that a great deal of psychological outreach is needed to maintain full awareness of the ups and downs of surgery. There is nothing wrong in being cognizant of life's contingencies, and in being ready to exercise our ability to strike our mental attitudes towards our intimal status of self-belief. Believing then becomes the positive, unstoppable force that will carry us through this and many other easy or complicated surgical feats.

Final Thoughts

I have given you and myself what I consider to be a worthwhile thought, a worthwhile attitude, and a worthwhile way of living: "Believe in yourself." This is, I think, one of the most important attitudinal changes we can embrace or maintain throughout our surgical and personal careers. Let's together make this a reality to reach a full and enhanced experience in surgery and in our lives. With this mental attitude, I can repeat, there will be no surgical case, within certain limits, which falls outside the scope of our cure. Let's do it!

References

1. Toledo-Pereyra LH. (1973) Galen's contribution to surgery. *Hist Med Allied Sci* **28**:357–375.
2. Toledo-Pereyra LH. (2007) Discovery according to Blalock. *J Invest Surg* **20**:145–147.
3. Toledo-Pereyra LH. (2007) The history of surgery according to Owen Wangensteen. *J Invest Surg* **20**:269–272.
4. Cooley DA. (1999) C. Walton Lillehei, the "Father of Open Heart Surgery." *Circulation* **100**:1364–1365.
5. Toledo-Pereyra LH. (ed.) (2007) *Reminiscences on Surgery, History and Humanities.* Landes Bioscience, Georgetown, TX.

19

Mentoring

by Luis H. Toledo-Pereyra, MD, PhD

Where Do We Start?

There is little question that mentoring begins when teaching is considered in the process of education. However, this is where the similarity ends since teaching remains more general, whereas mentoring is more specific or applied to an individual instead of a classroom. Teaching, therefore, requires mainly presentation skills whereas mentoring is more complex and long-term in essence.

Mentoring begins when an interested mentee and a committed mentor meet in common accordance.[1-12] Both need to exercise unwritten rules of mentoring that allow them to communicate with each other and to participate in common and agreed-upon goals. Where does mentoring start then? A plain answer might be that the relationship begins at the moment that the two parties accept to work with each other and recognize the importance of this educational or animic binary combination. The relationship starts at this moment, not before or not after. Understanding, accepting and working with mentoring is not that easy and, thus, requires intense interest and formal desire from both parties, that is, continuous commitment for both of them.

What is Mentoring?

Roget's Thesaurus Dictionary, under the term *mentor*, describes a *person who advises*, and then lists a series of nouns, such as *adviser, coach, counselor, guide, instructor, teacher, trainer, tutor*.[1] All of these names are good, but do not capture the essence of what I consider to be a mentor. For me, being a mentor or mentoring has a completely different connotation, and let me explain what I mean.

A mentor is a dedicated educator who represents and works with the mentee at frequent intervals to reach specific goals with defined timetables. The mentor is an intricate part of the mentee's dreams and professional aspirations. The mentor works often with the mentee to reach well-established guidelines and to prepare value-oriented work. The mentee is on the mind and expectations of the mentor, as both are looking for each other and seeking for similar academic pursuits.

In the surgical arena, the surgeon-mentor would need to include in the regular mentoring function the operating room (OR) setting, where mentoring becomes more defined and highly structured. The surgical principles in the OR should be clearly presented when mentoring occurs under these conditions. Qualities of patience, respect and understanding are essential to the surgeon-mentor's/surgical resident-mentee's long-lasting and positive relationship. Of all the desirable surgeon-mentor's virtues, perhaps the most important would be respect, which permits a constructive mentor-to-mentee affinity and the opportunity for establishing a durable communication path between the two of them.

Wiley Souba, in his well-researched paper on *Mentoring Young Academic Surgeons, Our Most Precious Asset*, published in 1999,[2] put forward a very precise and telling definition of a mentor. He wrote, "A mentor is someone who takes a special interest in helping another person (a mentoree) develop into a successful person." This is a short but especially pertinent explanation. The relationship emphasizes the interest of one person for another; carries a serious responsibility as to participating in the success of another person; implies a full compromise of the mentor towards the mentee. I would say that adding one more thing might make this compromise more comprehensive, and that is the commitment of the mentee towards the process of mentoring, where both the mentor and the mentee become fully engaged.

Who is a Good Mentor?

Being a good mentor is not a simple task, since it requires a long list of virtues acquired by the mentor and shared with the mentee, who reciprocally responds to this respectful association. As indicated previously, of all virtues or qualities it would be important to highlight respect, time, commitment, trust, determination, encouragement, patience, and opportunity for the mentee's independence as the fundamental characteristics of a good and reliable mentor. To the measure that all virtues are followed, the strength or capability of the mentor increases proportionally. The best mentors are the ones possessing all the virtues previously enumerated.

The mentee needs to search for a good mentor and all will depend on whether a good mentor is being searched for in the clinical arena, the research enterprise or the administrative side, or various combinations of these. The good mentor is not difficult to encounter if we train our faculty to become more participatory, willing to share their qualities and ability to communicate with others and be part of their academic lives.

A good mentor has a primary function of representing his/her mentee, being part of educational and research endeavors and offering wise advice when required. A good mentor is always there when there to help or advance the educational or professional goals of the mentee. A good mentor is always available. A good mentor responds immediately to the request of the disciple. A good mentor is an intricate part of the mentees' life and goals in academics and practice.

Who is a Good Mentee?

A good mentee is someone who effectively communicates and follows the wise advice of the mentor, who has academic and professional goals as his/her best objectives in mind. As the mentee advances in his/her career it is imperative that communication and follow-up remain at the center stage of their relationship. A good mentee is not possible without a good mentor. Likewise, a good mentor cannot exist without a good mentee.

The good mentee enjoys and frequently thrives in the presence of a good mentor. It is here, that both of them, a good mentor and a good mentee, re-ignite their lives together and learn how to maximize their fruitful relationship, a relationship of trust, support and respect. This is a relationship of understanding and goal-oriented aims, of mutual admiration and clear comprehension: a full relationship!

The Importance of a Good Mentor

There is no doubt about the importance of a good mentor since the mentor-mentee relationship is of paramount significance. A good mentor brings about the continuation of good practice, good professionalism, good research, good patient care, and ultimately a good individual worthy of being part of the career of choice.

It should be a great honor for the good mentor to be a special component of the life and functions of the mentee. The good mentor receives the confidence of the mentee and in response helps to mold his/her life in the best way possible. The good mentor is entrusted with the professional aspirations of the young and searching mentee. The good mentor actively participates in building new lives to be, at some point, an important section of the rich frame of society, the society we want and dream for future generations of productive professionals and individuals, a society worth belonging to.

A Clear Example of Mentoring

As I was reading my local newspaper, I came across an uplifting story of mentoring that I must pass along as a way to focus on the significance of a good mentor in life and medicine. The following is from the *Kalamazoo Gazette* printed on Friday, January 2, 2009.

> "When Trevor Banka treats cancer patients alongside Michael Mott, he not only is working with a man he calls his mentor but with the physician who helped save his life.
>
> "I wanted to work next to Dr. Mott and I wanted to train with him," said Banka, a 28-year-old second-year oncology resident at Detroit's Henry Ford Hospital. "We have a very special relationship."

That relationship started in 1993 when a 12-year-old Banka was diagnosed with bone cancer in his right knee.

Mott and his former partner performed the surgery, removing the cancerous bone and replacing Banka's knee with a prosthetic.

Mott continued to treat his patient throughout high school, college and even periodically while Banka attended medical school at Michigan State University.

Shortly after Banka joined Henry Ford, Mott transferred to the hospital. They now work together occasionally.

"He's very thorough and very meticulous," Banka said recently. "He has great technique. It's fun being on the other side of the stethoscope, being his patient and being his colleague."

Mott said some of his former patients have gone on to become nurses or physical therapists, but Banka is the only one who moved into oncology.

"Every now and then, he would say, 'I might do this stuff,'" said Mott, 45. "It certainly takes a lot of hard work and dedication, and he had to come up with all that on his own. He's a remarkable individual in that regard." — by Corey Williams

As this story unfolds, I realize the incredible impact of mentoring in medicine or surgery or the rest of the professions or jobs in the world. It is as if mentoring is the most coveted and pursued activity in our lives.

Mentoring as a Core Mission

In a recent paper, in 2007, Chandran and Bickel[3] reviewed the importance of considering mentoring as a core mission. They advanced the notion that "mentoring represents the most tangible bridge to continuing traditions of excellence and for succession planning." They wrote: "Because assessment drives performance and because mentoring is a crucial professional activity requiring great commitment and competency, medical schools are searching for ways to recognize and evaluate this as a core academic responsibility."[3]

It is obvious, then, that mentoring is at the crossroads of promoting and advancing the medical and surgical ideals of our profession. Without mentoring, our medical schools will lose their ability to train competent professionals, who in many ways embody the soul of our academic medical life. Mentoring conveys the essence of being to the physician and surgeon. Mentoring gives historical sense to the profession, and should be recognized as the real core mission of medicine and surgery.[4-12]

Mentoring in the Operating Room

The OR has a completely different atmosphere and standards from any other setting in medicine. It has well-defined principles and extremely well-characterized rules. In spite of that, tension is not an infrequent visitor and episodes of rush and anxiety become familiar. Under these conditions, mentoring requires well-prepared and particularly tolerant surgical minds.

A surgeon-mentor in the operating room is different from the surgeon-mentor outside the suite. The same surgeon can act differently when he/she is in or out of the OR. Therefore, special consideration should be given to creating the best atmosphere possible even under severe stress. There are no rules one can expect or readily follow except for rules of common sense and kind understanding.

How can one become a good mentor in the OR then? Even though this is a difficult question to answer, I would like to offer some ideas in this regard. The surgeon-mentor in the OR needs to be knowledgeable, respectful, patient, kind, generous and understanding. Following these qualities or traits of character, the surgeon-mentor should provide for the development of an amiable professional setting. That is the OR that one can aspire to create as the ideal place for the surgeon-mentor to teach and the surgeon-mentee to learn.

The surgeon-mentor of today should be different from the surgeon-mentor of yesterday. Besides knowledge and technique, respect and kindness are the essentials of a good surgeon-mentor master. Surgical training programs need to educate the faculty to be responsible to the principles outlined earlier. Surgeon-mentors need to exceed in patience and understanding to teach young surgeons the intricacies of the realm of surgery. Surgeon-mentors need to balance the teaching of surgical techniques within a spirit of kindness and humanism — a spirit of positive understanding where the new surgeons trained under these parameters will represent the best surgeons of the future.

Personal Reflections

As a surgical mentee, there are many surgeons whom I am indebted to because of their generous contributions to my development as a surgeon and as a human being. I can start in Huatabampo, Sonora, Mexico, where Dr. Victor Manuel Romo Ruiz kindly took me under his wing to show me the wonders of surgery while I was a young high school student. When off on vacation, I would impatiently await for Dr. Romo's highly regarded call. His message would represent an invitation to assist him in the OR. Dr. Romo was the ideal surgeon–mentor, patient, kind, respectful, understanding and willing to teach at any time all the concepts of critical importance in the OR. He was a great example to follow, someone who left a significant impression on me at my tender and inexperienced age.

My second exposure to a superior surgeon-mentor was in Mexico City at the end of medical school while doing my rotation, pregraduate internship at Juarez Hospital. The surgeon-mentor was Dr. Gilberto Lozano Saldivar, a man of principle and commitment to all interns and residents at the institution. Dr. Lozano brought class, knowledge and desire to teach into the OR. I learned a great deal from this excellent surgeon-mentor.

My third and longest exposure to an effective surgeon-mentor was during my surgical residency at the University of Minnesota. Dr. John S. Najarian represented a committed surgeon-master who was readily available whenever solicited. The coffee room in the premises but outside the OR on the fourth floor constituted his main center of action. If you required something, you knew where he was. His presence was evident and always attentive to the activities of faculty and trainees of the department. His approach was more of providing independence and full freedom to all of us who were commencing our surgical careers. As a surgeon-mentee, I found his mentoring techniques very unique as trust and understanding were essential to his practice of mentoring. I advanced a great deal by following these great opportunities.

On the other side of my surgical professional life, as a surgeon-mentor myself, I utilized my previous experiences to mold my teaching and mentoring capabilities. I began early during my surgical residency at Minnesota mentoring two close colleagues of mine, Javier Castellanos from Mexico City and Roberto Tersigni from Rome, Italy. During their surgical research experience in pancreas transplantation, I cherished having had the chance to work with them, advise them in planning specific projects, carry through, obtain the data, write the papers for publication and finally get all of them published. If publication was the main goal of this mentoring endeavor, I believe we were very successful.

As I advanced in my surgical life, I was fortunate enough to be exposed to a great number of talented surgeon-mentees. Many of them came from foreign countries and went back to make a significant imprint in surgery and in the local environment where they were practicing. My goal was to offer the best atmosphere possible for the young surgeon-mentee who came to our transplant and surgical research services. Basically, from 1977 when I started as surgical faculty at Henry Ford Hospital, then at Mount Carmel Mercy Hospital, both in Detroit, to Kalamazoo Borgess Medical Center, where I concluded my services in 2008, I proudly served dozens of surgical mentees for 31 years with the same principles of caring for their well-being and offering to them the best opportunity to learn the basics of the art and science of surgery.

In conclusion, the fundamentals of mentoring are based on mutual trust between the mentor and the mentee, as well as on the presence of respect, understanding and support. Both of them establish a covenant directed at maximizing the mentee's opportunities of progress in the field of their discipline. Mentor and mentee are equally responsible for a successful and fruitful endeavor.

References

1. *Roget's Thesaurus in Dictionary Form*. Second Edition. (1999) Princeton Language Institute, New York.
2. Souba WW. (1999) Mentoring young academic surgeons, our most precious asset. *J Surg Res* **82**:113–120.
3. Chandran L, Bickel J. (2007) Acting as if mentoring were a core mission. *Acad Phys Scient*: 7.

4. Detsky AS. (2007) Academic mentoring — how to give it and how to get it. *JAMA* **297**:2134–2136.

5. Lee JM, Anzai Y, Langlotz CP. (2006) Mentoring the mentors: aligning mentor and mentee expectations. *Acad Radiol* **13**:556–561.

6. Ramani S, Gruppen L, Kachur EK. (2006) Twelve tips for developing effective mentors. *Med Teach* **28**:404–408.

7. Singletary SE. (2005) Mentoring surgeons for the 21st century. *Ann Surg Oncol* **12**:848–860.

8. Hoover EL. (2005) Mentoring surgeons in private and academic practice. *Arch Surg* **140**:598–608.

9. Luna G. (2007) Mentoring the general surgeon. *Am J Surg* **193**:543–546.

10. Sambunjak D, Straus SE, Marusic A. (2006) Mentoring in academic medicine: a systematic review. *JAMA* **296**:1103–1115.

11. Freischlag JA. (2003) My mode of mentoring. *Surgery* **134**:416–417.

12. Musunnuru S, Lewis B, Rikkers LF, Chen H. (2007) Effective surgical residents strongly influence medical students to pursue surgical careers. *J Am Coll Surg* **204**:164–167.

20

Gentleman Surgeon

by Luis H. Toledo-Pereyra, MD, PhD

Centuries ago, being a gentleman surgeon meant having a status higher than the barber surgeon and the chirurgeon as well.[1-4] The gentleman surgeon was an educated and sophisticated surgeon who had learned from fellow gentlemen surgeons and had studied from books and in well-accepted centers of knowledge. Even though this surgeon was a great professional worth imitating, I am not referring to the individual surgeon's knowledge but to his/her personal qualities, that is, the behaviors that demonstrate caring, respect, and help for other fellow surgeons and patients in the development of the discipline. This is the gentleman surgeon who we will describe in this writing.

The Gentleman Surgeon Who Cares

For this philosophical review, the gentleman surgeon who cares is an individual who dedicates full attention and capability to the art and science of surgery, who advances the discipline in the best way possible, and who fully participates or engages in the betterment of this uplifting field of medicine.

The gentleman surgeon who cares commits to improving the treatment of patients throughout the entire evolution of the disease. The gentleman surgeon is characterized not only by advancing the knowledge of the malady in question, but by how much he/she is able to provide towards the care of the suffering person. Caring follows not only the body but the soul of the patient, caring understands the concerns and effects of disease in the affected individual, and shows full compassion towards the healing of the whole human being.

The gentleman surgeon who cares progresses in the specialty by advancing treatment for the ailments of the faltering human organism, defining why it is important to cure, and acknowledging separately the positive role of healing as compared to the technical characterization of treating. Dealing with the ill person, curing those who are suffering and promoting the human essence of the individual are the essential traits of the gentleman surgeon.

Not all great teaching surgeons necessarily show all the characteristics of the caring professional. Being a leading surgeon in the field does not automatically translate into being someone who cares. Caring is more complicated and is not part of the pioneering role of the surgeon. Undoubtedly, however, caring could advance the field to the highest level if applied in tandem with pioneering. They could handsomely supplement each other to the benefit of the patient and, of course, the surgeon as well.

The Gentleman Surgeon Who Respects

Respect for fellow surgeons, trainees, surgical personnel, and patients is an important component of the gentleman surgeon. This kind of professional offers consistent paths to recognize those who need respect, and understands how respect should be offered to them. The gentleman surgeon who respects brings to the surgical branch of medicine a unique opportunity for surgeon and patient improvement. He/she allows for better communication and understanding among all surgeons and patients.

It would be accurate enough to believe that respect unites surgeon, trainee and patient to better respond and appreciate their relationship and commitment to surgical matters. As well-defined as respect is, surgeons should endeavor to give building an environment of respect a top priority. We characterized respect before, in the following manner:[5]

> "Respect is the engine that supports human behavior. Without respect, civilizations would crumble. Individuals, therefore, require

respect to maintain society's interactions. The surgical world is not that different from society. Surgeons work and live within the norms and principles of respect. Respect for their fellow surgeons, for the operating room personnel and environment, and, of course, for patients and hospital activity is essential."

The gentleman surgeon who respects offers a positive environment where all — surgeons, trainees and patients alike — benefit by a special bond of common acceptance and mutual understanding. The gentleman surgeon who respects adds a new dimension to the operating room since the atmosphere is uplifting and well-worth experiencing. The gentleman surgeon who respects is admired and appreciated by all, including residents, fellows, nurses and administrators alike. There is no substitute for respect, just as there is no substitute for performing a good surgery while taking care of the patient in the operating theater.

The Gentleman Surgeon Who Helps

The gentleman surgeon who helps represents the ideal surgeon since spontaneous and well-intended support will always be well received and worth accepting. The gentleman surgeon who helps is an individual who engages in clinical practice, teaching, and research, since these areas of professional attention allow him/her to interact with the entire surgical team, and at the same time permit new opportunities for transforming the discipline.

In helping, you give. You enhance the chances of others as much as you help yourself. It is in helping others that you help yourself and test your real self-worth. The gentleman surgeon who helps is utilizing that unique time in his/her professional career to support others in the profession.

There are good examples in surgical history dealing with surgical pioneers who helped their students to help themselves, and at the same time created an enhanced surgical environment for the benefit of those practicing in this noble and worthwhile field of medicine. Try to help those in need in the profession: fellows, students, operating room personnel, recovery floor nurses. This will produce an improved attitude and a desire to be better and more focused in their work. The principle that I can see developing is "help others and they will help you." Even if that is not the case,

"Help others and you will help humanity, which in turn will help you." Better yet, "Help others regardless of the outcome." In this way the gentleman surgeon who helps will have a more fruitful and estimable life, one that would serve as a clear illustration for new generations to emulate.

Historical Representation of the Gentleman Surgeon Who Cares, Respects and Helps

The history of surgery can be an excellent guide for showing us the great discoveries of the discipline, leading us to the sources of those advances, and characterizing the evolution of the field. In as much as surgical history studies the evolution of the profession, historical accounts do not always investigate the virtues and character of its main performers.

Let me start by considering some of the giants of our profession to see how they shaped the surgical arena as far as the gentleman surgeon is concerned. Several names come to mind when analyzing those great surgical performers. Beginning in the latter part of the 19th century and first half of the 20th century, they are William Halsted (1852–1922) from Hopkins in Baltimore, Evarts Graham (1883–1957) from Washington University in St. Louis, and Owen Wangensteen (1898–1981) from the University of Minnesota in Minneapolis. Many others are deserving, but I would need an extensive writing to do justice to the volume of their accomplishments and their lives, and thus I will not be able to mention them here.[6–12]

We are not describing the surgeons' pioneering medical or surgical contributions at this point, but rather their gentleman surgeon capabilities as far as caring, respecting and helping. Halsted, Graham and Wangensteen, although from different eras and geographical locations, all believed in caring, respecting and helping. Because of the few descriptions available pertaining to their character, we need to use whatever has been written in analyzing their virtues and personalities.[8–10]

In the case of Halsted, we have the excellent description of his noted student, Harvey Cushing (1869–1939), father of American neurosurgery, who reviewed the character of his recognized mentor. Cushing pointed out the qualities and defects of his trusted tutor.[11] He saw Halsted as reserved, shy and reticent, and sometimes as taciturn and withdrawn, but in no instance did Halsted convey lack of caring, or disrespectful behavior, even though at times he could exhibit elements of sarcastic conduct. Overall, Professor Halsted commanded a great deal of respect, and at the same time he gave respect back to students and fellows.

In the case of Graham, his personality reflected his caring attitude and that of a gentleman surgeon who wanted to help faculty, trainees and students. Graham provided respect to associates and fellows as well. Graham was attentive to the needs of his staff and surgical team.[12] He considered no matter minimal or without importance. He was the ideal gentleman surgeon who cared, respected and helped others.

Regarding Wangensteen, his surgical fellows left a well-defined history alluding to his superb qualities as a gentleman surgeon in his professional life.[12] Many of Wangensteen's disciples spoke fondly about the master's extraordinary ability to care, respect and help his Minnesota students.[12] Richard Edlich, one of the younger, distinguished Wangensteen disciples characterized his beloved teacher very well when he wrote:[18]

> "Dr. Wangensteen had often told me that the chief responsibility of heads of department was to…create an atmosphere friendly to learning. He then said he must have the willingness to recognize every type of talent and ability and encourage people of promise. He must be the professor of the open door, easily accessible to his students, residents, and his associates."

Edlich continued to express that doctor Wangensteen supported his disciples all the way through; "realizing that the graduates' journey to success in teaching can be a tortuous one, he remained available to them for guidance and advice."[8] What an excellent way to summarize the attitude of Dr. Wangensteen as a gentleman surgeon who cared, respected and helped others in surgery.

Conclusion

The gentleman surgeon of today should possess three main characteristics. He/she cares, respects, and helps. These particular attitudes will project surgery to a humanistic level of unexpected and positive proportions. The surgeon-in-training, and later on the staff surgeon, should reach for means to become a gentleman surgeon with the qualities expressed above.

References

1. Toledo-Pereyra LH. (2006) *A History of American Medicine from the Colonial Period to the Early Twentieth Century.* The Edwin Mellen Press, Lewiston, NY.
2. Bell JB. (1975) *The Colonial Physician.* Science History Publications, NY.
3. Beck JB. (1850) *Medicine in the American Colonies.* Horn and Wallace Publishers, NY.
4. Toledo-Pereyra LH. (2006) Origins of surgery in British Colonial America. *J Invest Surg* **16**:3.
5. Toledo-Pereyra LH. (2005) Respect. *J Invest Surg* **18**:281–284.
6. Peltier LP, Aust JB. (1994) *L'Etoile Du Nord. An Account of Owen Harding Wangensteen (1898–1981).* American College of Surgeons, Chicago, IL.
7. MacCullum WG. (1930) *William Stewart Halsted, Surgeon.* John Hopkins Press, Baltimore, MD.
8. Edlich RF. (2007) In memoriam: a tribute to Dr. Owen H. Wangensteen, the greatest teacher of surgery during the 20th century (1898–1981). *J Surg Res* **138**:241–253.
9. Toledo-Pereyra LH. (2007) The history of surgery according to Owen Wangensteen. *J Invest Surg* **20**:269–272.
10. Meuller CB. (2002) *Evarts A. Graham: The Life, Lives, and Times of the Surgical Spirit of St. Louis.* Decker, Hamilton, BC.
11. Cushing H. (1922) In memoriam. William Stewart Halsted. *Science* **546**:461.
12. Najibi S, Frykberg ER. (2000) Owen H. Wangensteen, MD, PhD. A surgical legend and the father of modern management of intestinal obstruction (1898–1981). *Dig Surg* **17**:653–659.

Acknowledgments

Chapters 1 to 4, 6, 7, 9, 10, and 12 to 20 and their figures originally appeared in the *Journal of Investigative Surgery*, for which Dr. Toledo-Pereyra serves as Editor-in-Chief. We thank Informa Healthcare USA, Inc., 52 Vanderbilt Ave., New York, NY, 10017, for permission to reprint the essays in book form.

Chapter 5 first appeared in *History of American Medicine from the Colonial Period to the Early Twentieth Century* (ISBN 10 0-7734-5530-2), published by The Edwin Mellen Press, PO Box 450, Lewiston, NY, 14092. It is reprinted here with permission.

Figure Legends and Acknowledgments

Section I

Chapter 2 — *De Humani Corporis Fabrica*, Vesalius.

Figure 2.1. Picture of Vesalius, age 28. Previously published in *Journal of Investigative Surgery*, 21:232–236, 2008. Obtained from Malley CD. Andreas Vesalius of Brussels 1514–1564, Berkeley, CA, 1964.

Chapter 3 — Figures previously published in *Journal of Investigative Surgery*, 21:302–310, 2008.

Figure 3.1. Painted portrait of Harvey. Maintained at Hunterian Collection, University of Glasgow. Obtained from Keynes G. *The Portraiture of William Harvey*. The Royal College of Surgeons of England, London, 1949.

Figure 3.2. Diagram of Galen's cardiovascular system research. Obtained from Singer C. *A Short History of Anatomy and Physiology from the Greeks to Harvey*. Dover Publications, NY, 1957, p. 61.

Figure 3.3. *Exercitatio Anatomica* book cover, as published in 1628. From Persaud TVN. *A History of Anatomy. The Post-Vesalian Era*. Charles C. Thomas Publisher, Springfield, IL, 1997.

Chapter 4 — Figures previously published in *Journal of Investigative Surgery*, 22:4–8, 2009.

Figure 4.1. Painted portrait of Leeuwenhoek by artist Jan Verkolje, currently at the Rijksmuseum, The Netherlands. Painted between 1670 and 1693, Doek Technique, 56 × 47.5 cm.

Figure 4.2. Microscope of Leeuwenhoek being held by an unidentified observer. Photograph.

Chapter 6 — Figures previously published in *Journal of Investigative Surgery*, 22:157–161, 2009.

Figure 6.1. Photograph of Bernard in later life. No date or source identified. Obtained from Wikipedia.com, accessed on April 27, 2009.

Figure 6.2. The Lesson of Claude Bernard (1889). Oil painting by Leon-Agustin L'hermitte (1844–1915). This is an artistic depiction of animal vivisection at the College of France. Currently maintained at the Paris Academy of Medicine. Obtained from Wikipedia.com, accessed on April 27, 2009.

Chapter 7

Figure 7.1. Display of instruments used for Bernard's research. Obtained from www.claude-bernard.co.uk/page22.htm, accessed on September 15, 2010.

Chapter 10 — Figures previously published in *Journal of Investigative Surgery*, 22:327–332, 2009.

Figure 10.1. Wilhelm Roentgen (1845–1923) at the Institute of Physics at the University of Munich in 1906.

Figure 10.2. Hand radiograph of Roentgen's wife in 1895.

Figure 10.3. Pieces of buckshot are seen in Prescott Butler's hand in 1896. Obtained by Michael Pupin.

Section II

Chapter 13 — Figures previously published in *Journal of Investigative Surgery*, 22:162–166, 2009.

Figure 13.1. Arpad G. Gerster (1848–1923). Photo courtesy: The Mount Sinai Archives.

Figure 13.2. Max Thorek (1880–1960). Photo courtesy: Thorek Hospital, Chicago.

Chapter 14 — Figure previously published in *Journal of Investigative Surgery*, 22(4):234–238, 2009.

Figure 14.1. Michael E. DeBakey (1908–2008) displaying an artificial heart at a 1966 press conference. Photo obtained from Academy of Achievement, Washington, DC, at www.achievement.org.

Chapter 15 — Figure previously published in *Journal of Investigative Surgery*, 23:72–78, 2010.

Figure 15.1. Christiaan N. Barnard (1925–2002). Obtained from two-heartsfilm.com.

Chapter 16 — Figure previously published in *Journal of Investigative Surgery*, 23:1–5, 2010.

Figure 16.1. Christiaan N. Barnard (1925–2002) in 1968 photo. Credit to AP.

Index